THE BRAIN FOOD COOKBOOK

Recipes Inspired by the MIND Diet

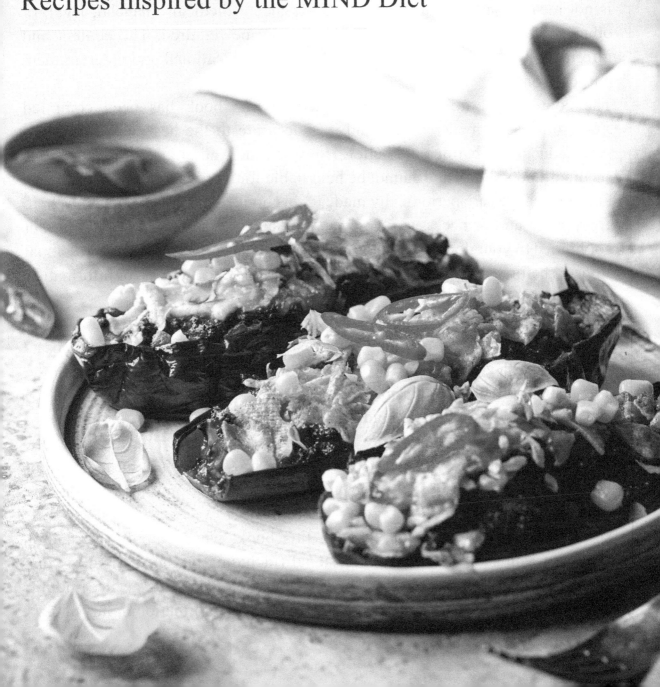

LEGAL & DISCLAIMER

The information contained in this book and its contents is not designed to replace or take the place of any form of medical or professional advice; and is not meant to replace the need for independent medical, financial, legal, or other professional advice or services, as may be required. The content and information in this book has been provided for educational and entertainment purposes only.

The content and information contained in this book has been compiled from sources deemed reliable, and it is accurate to the best of the Author's knowledge, information, and belief. However, the Author cannot guarantee its accuracy and validity and cannot be held liable for any errors and/or omissions. Further, changes are periodically made to this book as and when needed. Where appropriate and/or necessary, you must consult a professional (including but not limited to your doctor, attorney, financial advisor, or such other professional advisor) before using any of the suggested remedies, techniques, or information in this book.

Upon using the contents and information contained in this book, you agree to hold harmless the Author from and against any damages, costs, and expenses, including any legal fees potentially resulting from the application of any of the information provided by this book. This disclaimer applies to any loss, damages or injury caused by the use and application, whether directly or indirectly, of any advice or information presented, whether for breach of contract, tort, negligence, personal injury, criminal intent, or under any other cause of action. You agree to accept all risks of using the information presented inside this book.

You agree that by continuing to read this book, where appropriate and/or necessary, you shall consult a professional (including but not limited to your doctor, attorney, or financial advisor or such other advisor as needed) before using any of the suggested remedies, techniques, or information in this book.

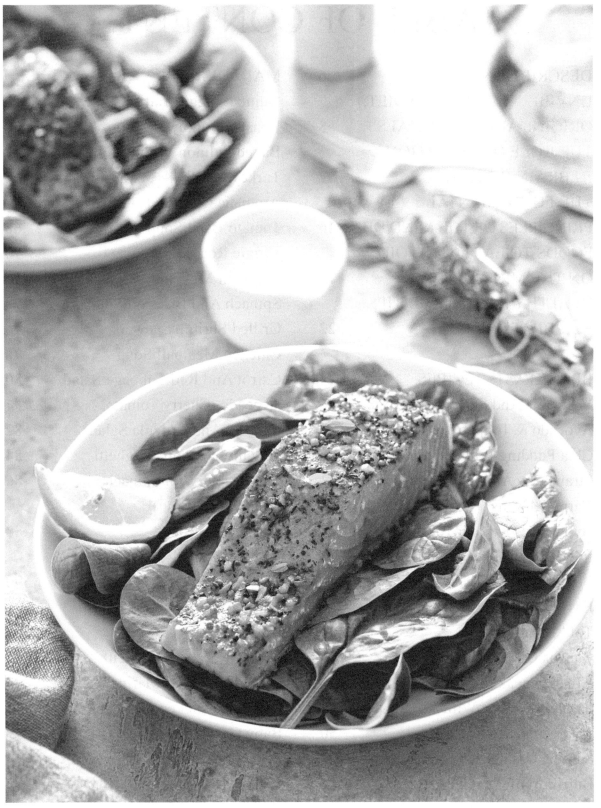

TABLE OF CONTENTS

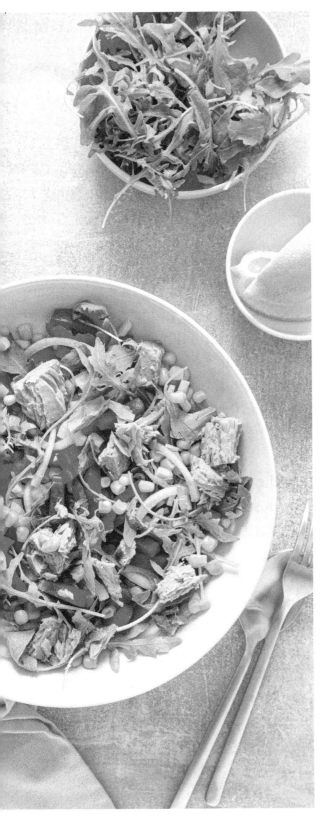

DESCRIPTION

Welcome to the world of the MIND Diet – an innovative diet developed based on scientific research aimed at supporting brain health. We are delighted to welcome you on the journey to improving your diet and, consequently, your health and well-being.

The brain is our most vital organ. It governs all aspects of our lives, from thoughts and feelings to movements and breath. It's no wonder that taking care of brain health is becoming increasingly important in our modern world, filled with stress, information overload, and not always optimal nutrition.

The MIND Diet (Mediterranean-DASH Intervention for Neurodegenerative Delay) is a unique combination of principles from the Mediterranean diet and the DASH diet (Dietary Approaches to Stop Hypertension), scientifically proven to improve brain health and reduce the risk of neurodegenerative diseases such as Alzheimer's and Parkinson's.

In this book, we not only present to you the principles and essence of the MIND Diet but also a wide array of delicious and nutritious recipes crafted in accordance with the diet's recommendations. You will learn which foods to include in your diet to support brain health and which dietary habits may lead to its deterioration.

The main goal of our book is to help you not only improve your nutrition but also do it in an enjoyable and tasty way. The journey to brain health can be a fun and flavorful adventure, and we invite you to join us on this exciting journey.

Let's explore the MIND Diet together and discover how its principles can transform your health and your life. Let's go!

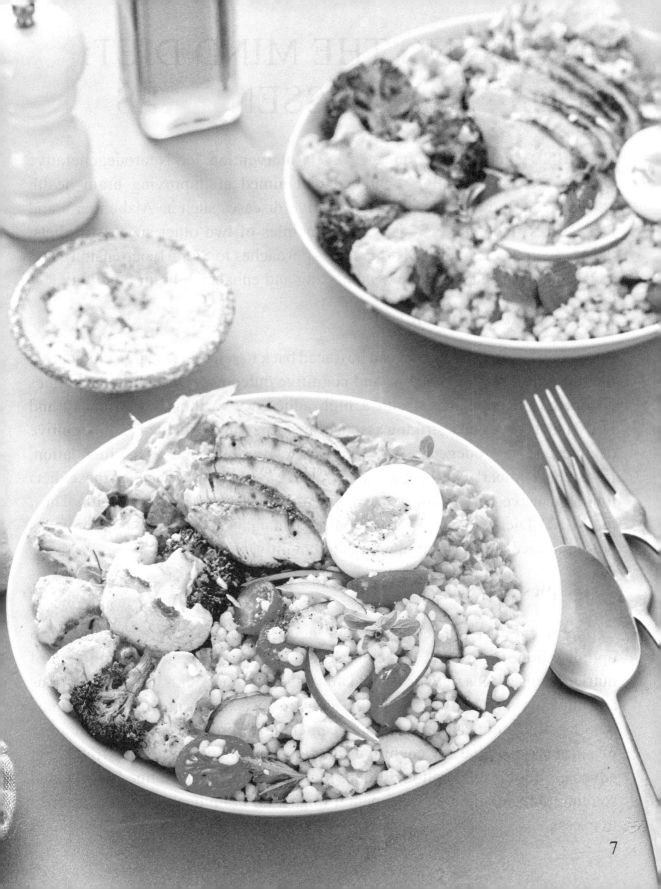

UNVEILING THE MIND DIET: ORIGINS AND ESSENTIALS

The MIND Diet (Mediterranean-DASH Intervention for Neurodegenerative Delay) is a scientifically researched diet aimed at improving brain health and reducing the risk of neurodegenerative diseases such as Alzheimer's and Parkinson's. This diet combines the principles of two other successful diets, the Mediterranean and DASH (Dietary Approaches to Stop Hypertension), and adds unique aspects focused on supporting and enhancing brain function.

Origins and Evolution

The genesis of the MIND Diet can be traced back to seminal research elucidating the link between dietary habits and cognitive outcomes. Observational studies conducted on populations with a high adherence to the Mediterranean and DASH diets revealed a striking association with reduced incidence of cognitive decline and neurodegenerative conditions. Building upon this foundation, researchers embarked on a quest to distill the essential elements of these diets into a cohesive framework tailored specifically to support brain health. Thus, the MIND Diet was born—a harmonious amalgamation of dietary principles poised to revolutionize our approach to cognitive wellness.

Principles and Pillars

Central to the MIND Diet are its guiding principles, meticulously crafted to optimize brain health and longevity. The diet emphasizes the consumption of nutrient-dense foods rich in antioxidants, omega-3 fatty acids, and key vitamins and minerals known to exert neuroprotective effects. Leafy greens, berries, nuts, whole grains, and lean proteins take center stage, providing a bountiful array of nutrients essential for cognitive function. Simultaneously, the MIND Diet advocates for the moderation of foods high in saturated fats, refined sugars, and sodium, recognizing their detrimental impact on brain health when consumed in excess.

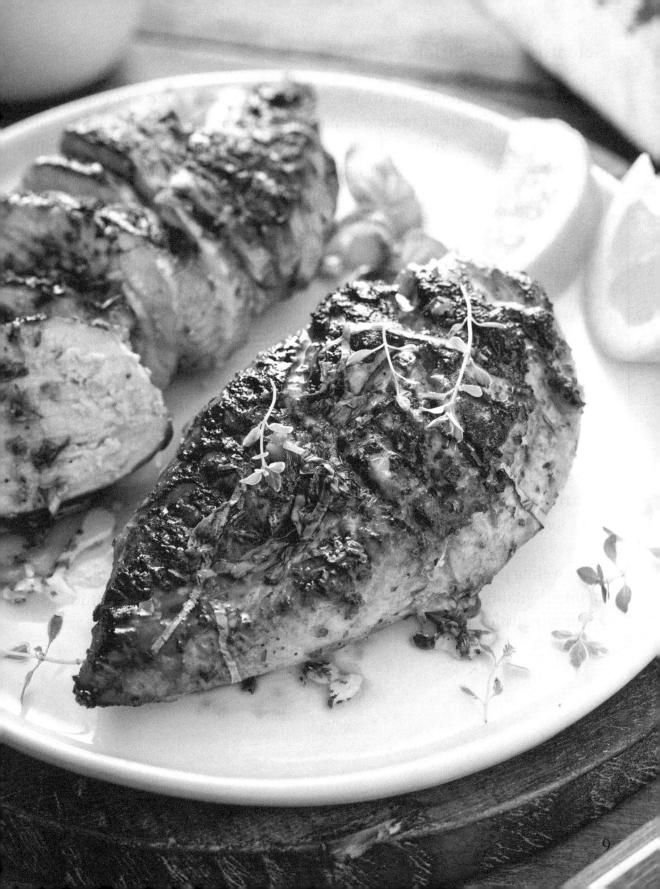

Scientific Foundation

The scientific underpinnings of the MIND Diet are robust and compelling, grounded in a wealth of research spanning epidemiology, neuroscience, and nutritional science. Studies have consistently demonstrated the profound influence of dietary patterns on brain structure and function, with adherence to the MIND Diet correlating with a lower risk of cognitive decline, dementia, and Alzheimer's disease. Mechanistic insights further elucidate the pathways through which specific nutrients exert their protective effects, shedding light on the intricate interplay between diet and brain health.

Empowering Dietary Choices

Armed with knowledge of the MIND Diet's principles and scientific rationale, individuals are empowered to make informed dietary choices that prioritize brain health and cognitive longevity. By adopting a pattern of eating rich in brain-boosting nutrients and mindful of potential pitfalls, individuals can embark on a journey towards optimal cognitive vitality and resilience. In the pages that follow, we delve deeper into the practical aspects of implementing the MIND Diet, providing guidance, recipes, and strategies to support your quest for cognitive wellness.

In unraveling the essence of the MIND Diet, we unlock the key to a future where cognitive vitality knows no bounds—a future shaped by the transformative power of nutrition and the unwavering commitment to brain health.

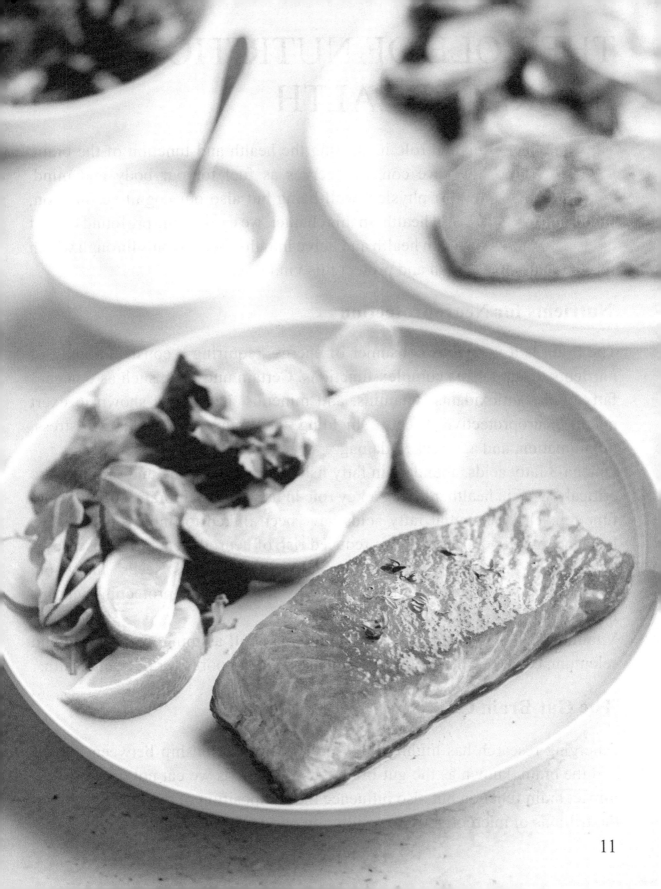

THE ROLE OF NUTRITION IN BRAIN HEALTH

Nutrition plays a pivotal role in shaping the health and function of the brain. Every morsel of food we consume serves as fuel for our body and mind, influencing not only our physical well-being but also our cognitive function, mood, and overall mental health. In this chapter, we explore the profound impact of dietary choices on brain health and delve into the mechanisms through which specific nutrients nourish and protect this vital organ.

Nutrients for Neuroprotection

The brain is a voracious consumer of energy, requiring a constant supply of nutrients to support its complex functions. Certain nutrients, such as omega-3 fatty acids, antioxidants, vitamins, and minerals, have been shown to exert potent neuroprotective effects, shielding the brain from oxidative stress, inflammation, and age-related damage.

Omega-3 fatty acids, abundant in fatty fish like salmon, trout, and sardines, are critical for brain health, playing a key role in neuronal membrane structure and function. These essential fatty acids have been linked to improved cognitive function, mood regulation, and a reduced risk of neurodegenerative diseases.

Antioxidants, found in colorful fruits and vegetables, nuts, seeds, and whole grains, combat oxidative damage caused by free radicals, protecting neurons from premature aging and degeneration.

Vitamins such as vitamin E and vitamin C, as well as minerals like zinc and selenium, contribute to antioxidant defenses and support overall brain health.

The Gut-Brain Connection

Emerging research has highlighted the intricate relationship between the gut and the brain, known as the gut-brain axis. The foods we eat not only directly impact brain function but also influence the composition of the gut microbiota, the trillions of microorganisms residing in our gastrointestinal tract.

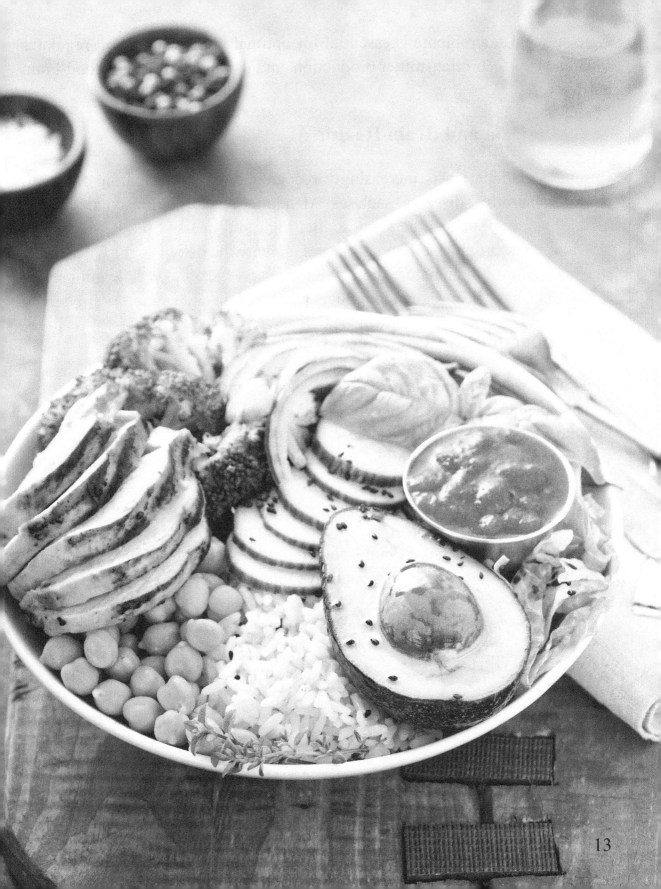

13

A healthy gut microbiome is essential for optimal brain health, as it regulates inflammation, neurotransmitter production, and the integrity of the blood-brain barrier.

Inflammation and Brain Health

Chronic inflammation is increasingly recognized as a contributing factor to neurodegenerative diseases such as Alzheimer's and Parkinson's. Certain dietary patterns, such as the Western diet high in processed foods, sugar, and unhealthy fats, promote inflammation and increase the risk of cognitive decline. In contrast, anti-inflammatory diets rich in fruits, vegetables, whole grains, and healthy fats have been shown to reduce inflammation and support brain health.

The Impact of Lifestyle Factors

In addition to nutrition, lifestyle factors such as physical activity, sleep, stress management, and social connections play a crucial role in brain health. A holistic approach that addresses these factors alongside dietary interventions is essential for preserving cognitive function and promoting overall well-being.

In summary, nutrition is a cornerstone of brain health, with specific nutrients and dietary patterns exerting profound effects on cognitive function and resilience. By prioritizing a diet rich in brain-boosting nutrients, individuals can nourish their minds and support lifelong cognitive vitality.

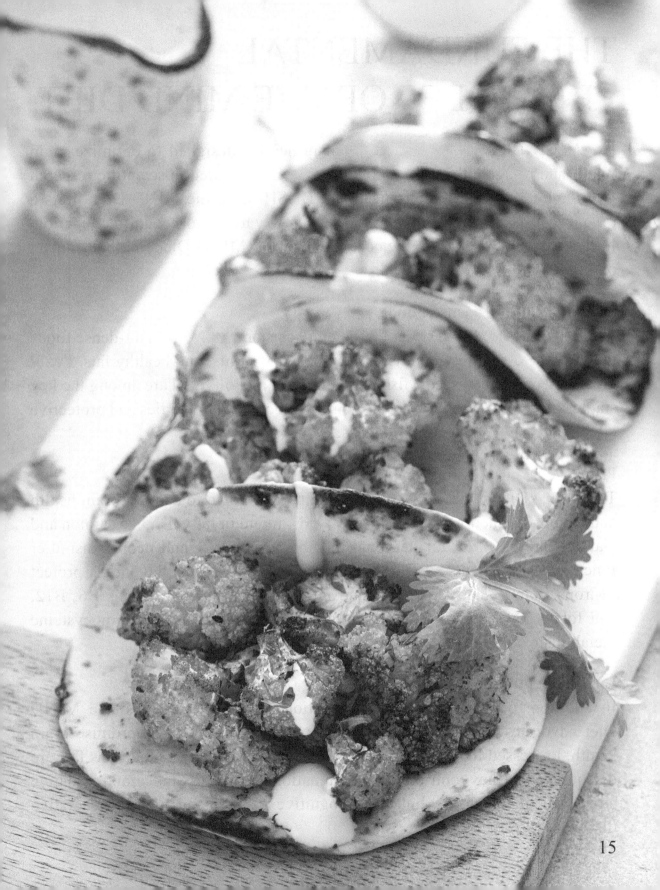

THE FUNDAMENTAL PRINCIPLES OF THE MIND DIET

The MIND Diet encapsulates a set of principles designed to optimize brain health and mitigate the risk of cognitive decline. Rooted in scientific research and inspired by the Mediterranean and DASH diets, the MIND Diet offers a unique approach to nutrition tailored specifically to support cognitive function. In this chapter, we explore the core tenets of the MIND Diet and their impact on brain health.

Embrace Nutrient-Dense Foods:
At the heart of the MIND Diet lies an emphasis on whole, nutrient-dense foods that provide essential vitamins, minerals, antioxidants, and healthy fats. Leafy greens, berries, nuts, seeds, fish, whole grains, and olive oil are among the key staples of the diet, chosen for their cognitive-boosting properties and protective effects against neurodegenerative diseases.

Prioritize Brain-Boosting Nutrients:
The MIND Diet places a premium on nutrients known to support brain health and cognitive function. Omega-3 fatty acids, found in fatty fish like salmon and walnuts, are essential for neuronal membrane integrity and neurotransmitter function. Antioxidants such as vitamin E, vitamin C, and flavonoids protect neurons from oxidative damage and inflammation, while vitamins B6, B12, and folate play crucial roles in neurotransmitter synthesis and homocysteine metabolism.

Limit Harmful Foods:
In addition to promoting the consumption of beneficial foods, the MIND Diet advocates for the restriction of substances that may compromise brain health. Processed foods high in refined sugars, saturated fats, and trans fats are discouraged, as they contribute to inflammation, insulin resistance, and oxidative stress, all of which are linked to cognitive decline and neurodegenerative diseases.

16

Embrace Moderation and Balance:

While certain foods are encouraged on the MIND Diet, moderation and balance are key principles guiding dietary choices. Portion control and mindful eating practices help prevent overconsumption of calorie-dense foods and promote a balanced intake of macronutrients. By striking a harmonious balance between indulgence and restraint, individuals can enjoy a varied and satisfying diet while supporting brain health.

Foster Consistency and Long-Term Adherence:

The MIND Diet is not a short-term fad but a sustainable lifestyle approach aimed at promoting lifelong brain health. Consistency and long-term adherence to the principles of the diet are essential for reaping its full benefits. By integrating the MIND Diet into daily life and making informed dietary choices, individuals can nourish their brains and safeguard cognitive function well into the future.

In summary, the MIND Diet offers a comprehensive framework for promoting brain health through nutrition, emphasizing the consumption of nutrient-rich foods, the restriction of harmful substances, and the cultivation of moderation and balance. By embracing these fundamental principles, individuals can harness the transformative power of diet to support cognitive vitality and enhance overall well-being.

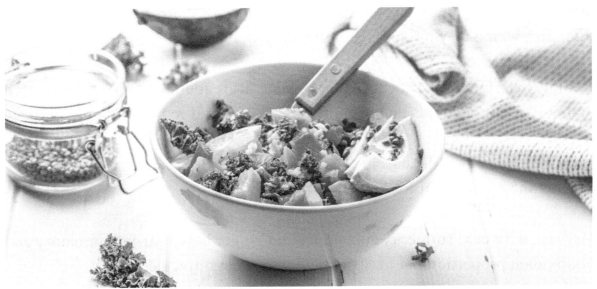

FOODS TO EAT AND AVOID ON THE MIND DIET

Foods to Eat:

Leafy Greens: Spinach, kale, collard greens, and Swiss chard are rich sources of vitamins, minerals, and antioxidants that promote brain health.

Berries: Blueberries, strawberries, raspberries, and blackberries are packed with antioxidants and flavonoids that protect against oxidative stress and inflammation in the brain.

Nuts and Seeds: Walnuts, almonds, flaxseeds, and chia seeds provide omega-3 fatty acids, vitamin E, and other nutrients essential for brain function.

Fatty Fish: Salmon, mackerel, trout, and sardines are excellent sources of omega-3 fatty acids, which have been shown to support cognitive function and reduce the risk of neurodegenerative diseases.

Whole Grains: Quinoa, brown rice, oats, and barley are rich in fiber and B vitamins, which play a role in cognitive function and mood regulation.

Healthy Fats: Olive oil, avocado, and coconut oil are sources of monounsaturated and polyunsaturated fats that support brain health and reduce inflammation.

Legumes: Beans, lentils, and chickpeas are high in fiber, protein, and antioxidants, making them beneficial for brain health.

Herbs and Spices: Turmeric, cinnamon, and ginger have anti-inflammatory and antioxidant properties that may protect against cognitive decline.

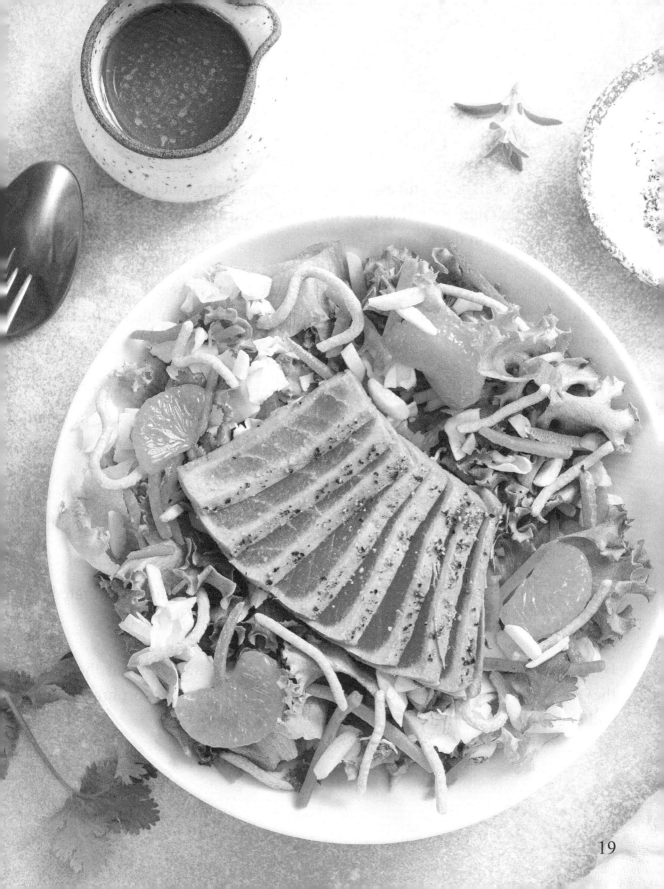

Foods to Avoid or Limit:

Processed Foods: Highly processed foods such as sugary snacks, refined grains, and fast food should be limited, as they can contribute to inflammation and insulin resistance in the brain.

Red and Processed Meat: Red meat and processed meats like bacon and sausage should be consumed sparingly, as they have been linked to an increased risk of cognitive decline.

Sweets and Desserts: Foods high in added sugars, such as candy, pastries, and soda, should be avoided or limited, as they can impair cognitive function and increase the risk of dementia.

Butter and Margarine: High-fat dairy products and hydrogenated oils should be limited, as they are sources of saturated and trans fats that can promote inflammation in the brain.

Cheese: While cheese can be consumed in moderation, it is high in saturated fat and sodium, so it should be enjoyed sparingly on the MIND Diet.

By following these guidelines and making mindful choices about the foods they eat, individuals can harness the power of nutrition to support brain health and cognitive function on the MIND Diet.

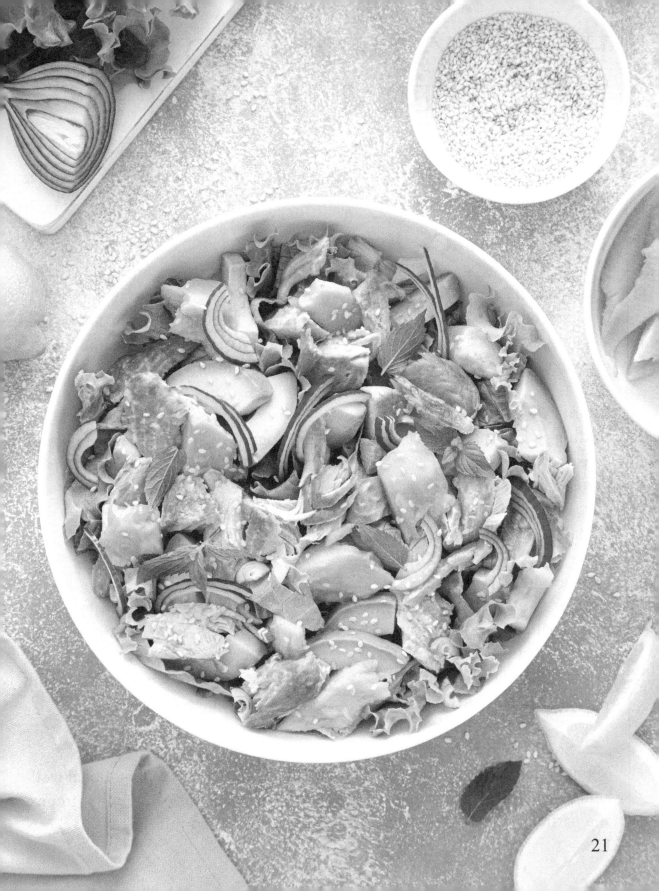

HEALTHY HABITS AND TIPS FOR BRAIN HEALTH

In this chapter, we delve into the importance of adopting healthy habits and incorporating brain-boosting strategies into daily life to support cognitive function and overall well-being.

Stay Physically Active:
Regular exercise is essential for brain health, as it improves blood flow to the brain, stimulates the production of growth factors that promote the growth of new neurons, and reduces the risk of cognitive decline. Aim for at least 30 minutes of moderate-intensity exercise most days of the week, incorporating a mix of aerobic exercise, strength training, and flexibility exercises.

Prioritize Quality Sleep:
Getting adequate sleep is crucial for cognitive function and memory consolidation. Aim for 7-9 hours of quality sleep each night, and establish a regular sleep schedule by going to bed and waking up at the same time each day. Create a relaxing bedtime routine, and avoid caffeine, electronics, and stimulating activities before bed to promote better sleep.

Manage Stress:
Chronic stress can have detrimental effects on brain health, contributing to inflammation, oxidative stress, and impaired cognitive function. Practice stress-reduction techniques such as deep breathing, meditation, yoga, or tai chi to promote relaxation and mental well-being. Engage in activities that bring you joy and fulfillment, and prioritize self-care to reduce stress levels.

Stay Socially Connected:
Maintaining social connections is essential for brain health and emotional well-being. Spend time with family and friends, join clubs or community groups, and participate in social activities that bring you joy and fulfillment.

22

Engage in meaningful conversations and cultivate supportive relationships to boost mood and cognitive function.

Challenge Your Brain:
Keep your brain active and engaged by challenging yourself with mentally stimulating activities. Try new hobbies, learn a new language, play brain games or puzzles, or engage in activities that require problem-solving and critical thinking skills. Stimulating your brain regularly can help build cognitive reserve and reduce the risk of cognitive decline as you age.

Follow a Brain-Healthy Diet:
Adopting a diet rich in brain-boosting nutrients is essential for optimal cognitive function and brain health. Follow the principles of the MIND Diet, which emphasizes the consumption of fruits, vegetables, whole grains, healthy fats, and lean proteins while limiting processed foods, saturated fats, and added sugars. Stay hydrated by drinking plenty of water throughout the day, as dehydration can impair cognitive function and mood.

Engage in Lifelong Learning:
Continuously challenging your mind through learning and education is a powerful way to promote cognitive health. Whether it's taking a class, attending workshops, reading books, or listening to podcasts on topics that interest you, exposing yourself to new ideas and information can stimulate neural connections, improve memory retention, and enhance cognitive flexibility.

Practice Mindfulness and Mindful Eating:
Mindfulness practices, such as meditation, deep breathing exercises, and mindful eating, can help reduce stress, improve focus, and enhance self-awareness. Incorporate mindfulness into your daily routine by taking moments to pause, breathe deeply, and cultivate present-moment awareness.

By incorporating these healthy habits and brain-boosting strategies into your daily routine, you can support cognitive function, enhance memory and concentration, and promote overall brain health and well-being.

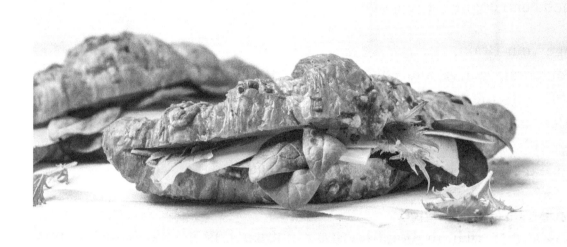

BREAKFAST RECIPES

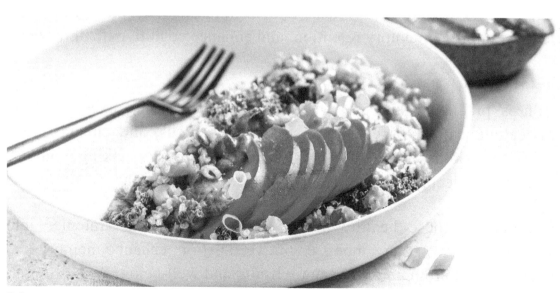

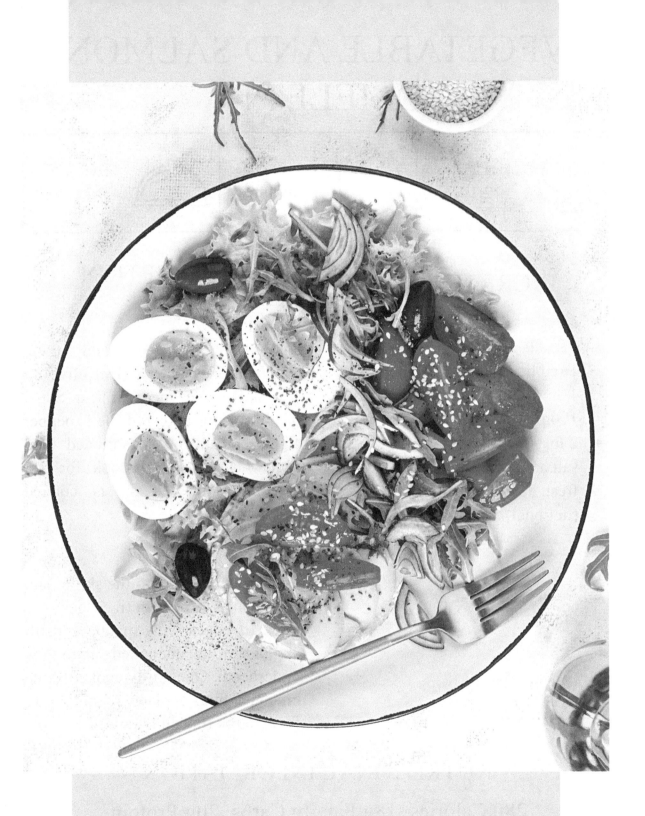

VEGETABLE AND SALMON OMELETTE

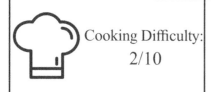 Cooking Difficulty: 2/10

 Cooking Time: 10 minutes

 Servings: 2

INGREDIENTS

- 4 eggs
- 1 small green onion, chopped
- 1 red bell pepper, chopped
- 1 small tomato, chopped
- 100g fresh salmon, diced
- 2 tbsp olive oil
- salt and pepper to taste
- fresh herbs for garnish (optional)

DESCRIPTION

STEP 1
Whisk eggs in a bowl and season with salt and pepper. Heat olive oil in a skillet over medium heat. Sauté green onion and red bell pepper for 3-4 minutes until softened. Add tomato and salmon, cook for 2-3 minutes until salmon is cooked through.

STEP 2
Pour beaten eggs into the skillet and stir gently. Cook until edges set, then lift edges with spatula and tilt skillet to allow uncooked egg to flow underneath. Once fully cooked, slide omelette onto a plate, garnish with fresh herbs if desired, and serve hot.

NUTRITIONAL INFORMATION

280 Calories, 18g Fat, 4g Carbs, 20g Protein

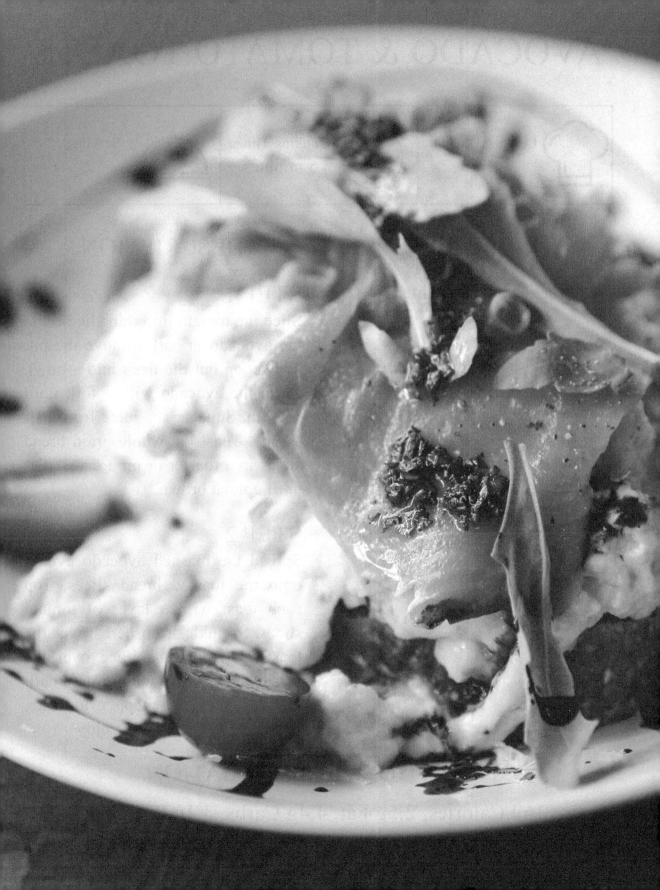

AVOCADO & TOMATO TOASTS

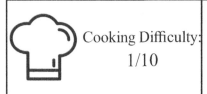 Cooking Difficulty: 1/10

 Cooking Time: 5 minutes

 Servings: 2

INGREDIENTS

- 2 slices whole grain bread
- 1 large avocado
- 1 large tomato
- juice of half a lime
- fresh herbs (such as cilantro or basil)
- ground chili powder to taste
- salt and pepper to taste

DESCRIPTION

STEP 1

Slice the tomato into thin slices. Cut the avocado in half, remove the pit, and scoop out the flesh into a bowl. Mash the avocado with a fork until smooth. Squeeze the juice from half a lime. Toast the whole grain bread slices in a toaster or on a dry skillet until golden brown.

STEP 2

Spread the mashed avocado evenly onto the toasted bread slices. Top each toast with a layer of tomato slices. Sprinkle fresh herbs over the toasts. Drizzle lime juice over the toasts and sprinkle with ground chili powder, salt, and pepper to taste. Serve the toasts hot and enjoy!

NUTRITIONAL INFORMATION

169 Calories, 2.5g Fat, 4.4g Carbs, 3.1g Protein

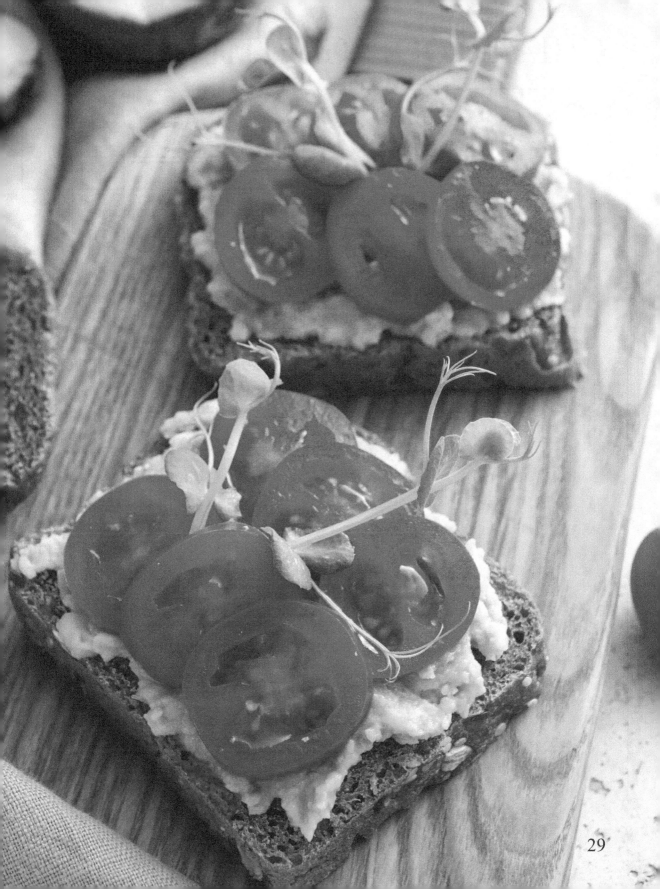

CHIA PUDDING WITH ALMOND

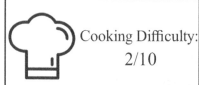 Cooking Difficulty: 2/10

 Cooking Time: 24 minutes

 Servings: 2

INGREDIENTS

- 4 tablespoons chia seeds
- 1 cup plant-based milk (such as coconut or almond milk)
- 2 tablespoons almond flakes
- 1/4 cup fresh or frozen blueberries
- 1/2 teaspoon vanilla extract
- natural honey or maple syrup to taste (optional)
- almond slices for garnish (optional)

DESCRIPTION

STEP 1
In a large bowl, mix chia seeds and plant-based milk. Add vanilla extract and stir well. Place the bowl in the refrigerator for 15-20 minutes to allow the pudding to thicken.

STEP 2
Once the pudding starts to thicken, remove it from the refrigerator and stir again to distribute the chia seeds evenly. Divide the chia pudding into two servings and top with almond flakes and blueberries.

STEP 3
Optionally, drizzle with natural honey or maple syrup for sweetness. Garnish with almond slices before serving.

NUTRITIONAL INFORMATION

210 Calories, 8g Fat, 10g Carbs, 5g Protein

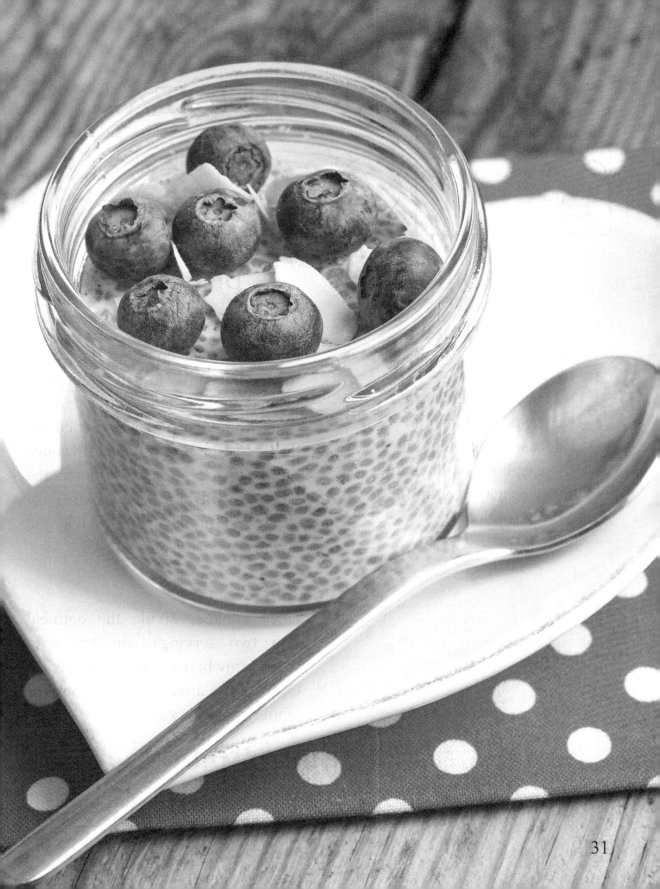

STRAWBERRY AND BLUEBERRY OATMEAL

 Cooking Difficulty: 2/10

 Cooking Time: 9 minutes

 Servings: 2

INGREDIENTS

- 1 cup rolled oats
- 2 cups oat milk
- 1/2 cup fresh strawberries
- 1/2 cup fresh blueberries
- 1/2 teaspoon cinnamon
- 1/4 teaspoon ground ginger
- 1/4 teaspoon vanilla extract
- honey or maple syrup for serving (optional)

DESCRIPTION

STEP 1
In a saucepan, combine the rolled oats and oat milk. Add the cinnamon, ground ginger, and vanilla extract. Bring to a gentle boil over medium heat, stirring occasionally. Reduce the heat to low and simmer the oatmeal, stirring occasionally, for about 5-7 minutes until thick and creamy.

STEP 2
Once cooked, divide the oatmeal into two servings and top with fresh strawberries and blueberries. Optionally, drizzle with honey or maple syrup for sweetness.

NUTRITIONAL INFORMATION

250 Calories, 5g Fat, 44g Carbs, 7g Protein

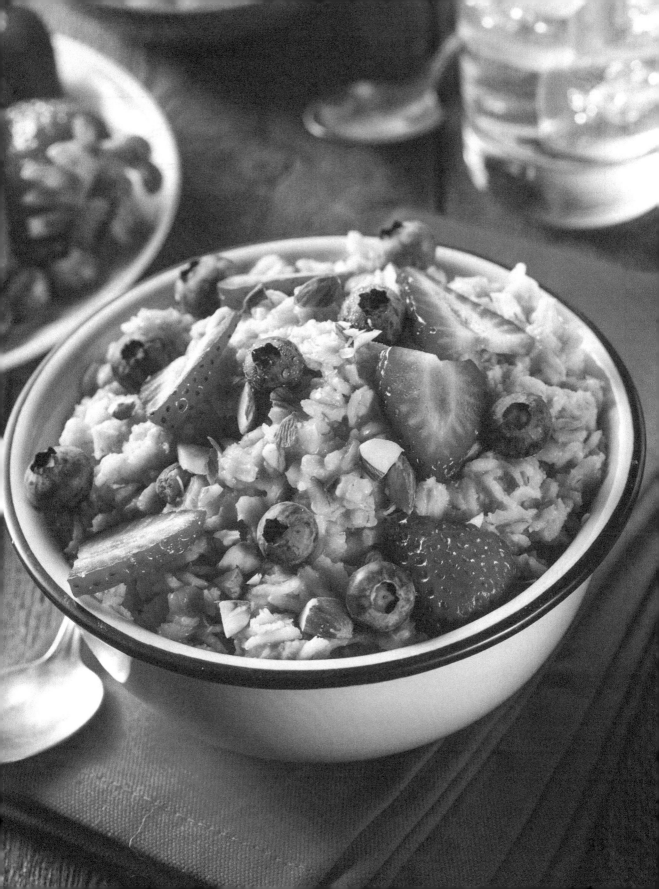

CARROT MUFFINS

 Cooking Difficulty: 3/10

 Cooking Time: 38 minutes

 Servings: 2

INGREDIENTS

- 1 1/2 cups all-purpose flour (or whole wheat flour)
- 1 cup grated carrots
- 1/2 cup honey or maple syrup
- 1/3 cup vegetable oil (such as coconut or olive oil)
- 2 eggs
- 1 teaspoon baking powder
- 1 teaspoon cinnamon
- 1/2 teaspoon ground ginger (optional)
- pinch of salt
- zest of an orange or lemon (optional)
- walnuts or raisins for garnish (optional)

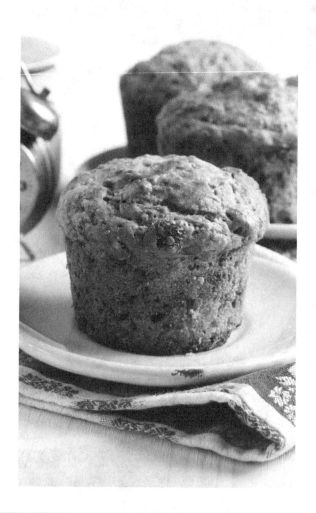

NUTRITIONAL INFORMATION

Calories: 180; Fat: 8 g; Carbs: 20 g; Protein: 3g

DESCRIPTION

STEP 1
Preheat the oven to 350°F (175°C). Line a muffin tin with paper liners.

STEP 2
In a large bowl, mix together the flour, baking powder, cinnamon, ground ginger (if using), and a pinch of salt.

STEP 3
In another bowl, beat the eggs with honey or maple syrup until smooth. Gradually add the vegetable oil, continuing to beat.

STEP 4
Gradually add the dry ingredients to the wet ingredients, gently stirring until you have a thick batter.

STEP 5
Fold in the grated carrots and orange or lemon zest (if using) until evenly distributed.

STEP 6
Pour the batter into the prepared muffin tin, filling each muffin cup about 2/3 full.

STEP 7
Garnish each muffin with walnuts or raisins (if using). Bake the muffins in the preheated oven for about 20-25 minutes, or until golden brown and a toothpick inserted into the center comes out clean.

STEP 8
Allow the muffins to cool in the tin for 5-10 minutes, then transfer them to a wire rack to cool completely. Serve.

AVOCADO & SALMON TOASTS

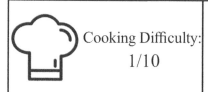 Cooking Difficulty: 1/10

 Cooking Time: 5 minutes

 Servings: 2

INGREDIENTS

- 2 slices whole wheat bread
- 1 large avocado
- 100g fresh salmon
- juice of half a lime
- salt and pepper to taste
- fresh herbs for garnish (such as cilantro or parsley)

DESCRIPTION

STEP 1

Cut the avocado in half, remove the pit, and scoop the flesh into a bowl. Mash the avocado with a fork until smooth. Add lime juice to the mashed avocado and mix well. Season with salt and pepper to taste.

STEP 2

Slice the fresh salmon into thin slices. Toast the slices of bread until golden brown. Spread the mashed avocado evenly onto the toasted bread slices. Arrange the slices of salmon on top of the avocado. Garnish with fresh herbs and season with additional salt and pepper if desired.

NUTRITIONAL INFORMATION

300 Calories, 18g Fat, 20g Carbs, 15g Protein

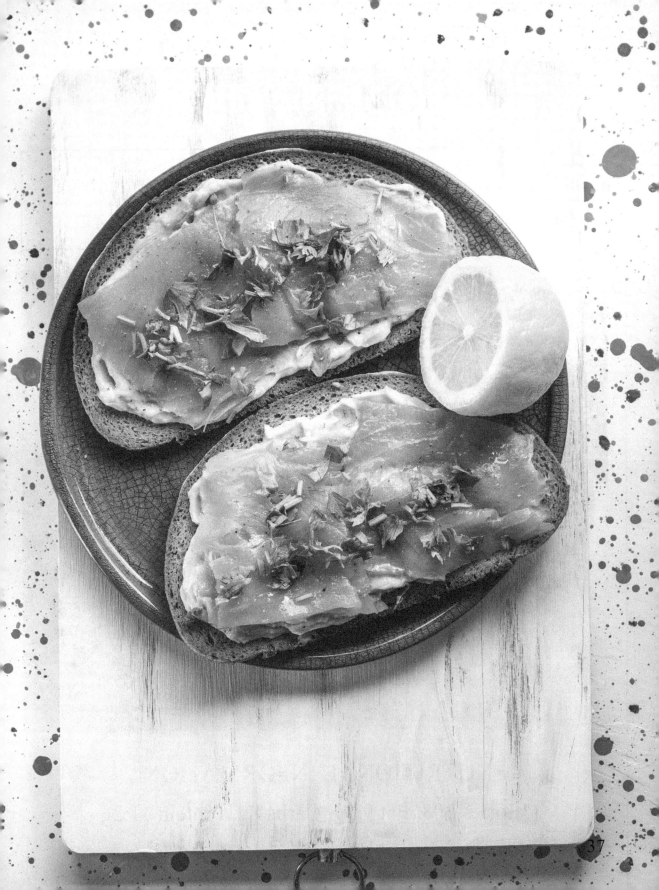

POTATO VEGETABLE OMELETTE

Cooking Difficulty: 2/10	Cooking Time: 18 minutes	Servings: 2

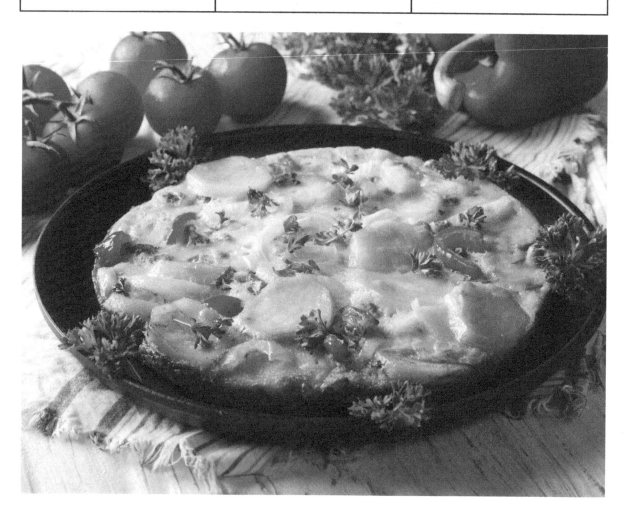

NUTRITIONAL INFORMATION

Calories 308, Fat 9.2g, Carbs 8g, Protein 11.2g

INGREDIENTS

- 2 medium potatoes
- 1 small onion
- 1 medium tomato
- 1 green bell pepper
- 4 eggs
- salt and pepper to taste
- fresh herbs for garnish (optional)

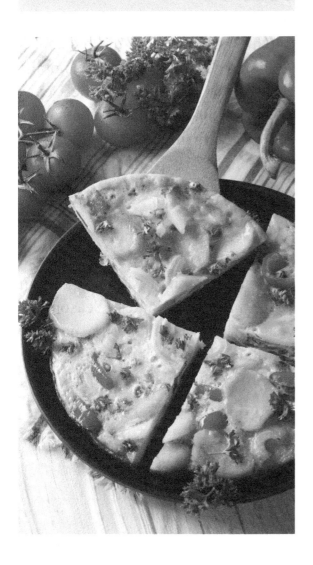

DESCRIPTION

STEP 1
Prepare the potatoes by slicing them into thin rounds or cubes. Dice the onion, tomato, and bell pepper into small pieces. Preheat the air fryer to 180 degrees Celsius (356 degrees Fahrenheit).

STEP 2
In a large bowl, beat the eggs and add the chopped vegetables, salt, and pepper. Mix thoroughly.

STEP 3
Evenly distribute the egg and vegetable mixture into a greased or parchment-lined baking dish.

STEP 4
Place the dish in the air fryer and cook at 356 degrees Fahrenheit for 10-12 minutes, or until the omelette is golden and firm.

STEP 5
Once the omelette is cooked, slice it into portions, garnish with fresh herbs if desired, and serve immediately. Enjoy your healthy breakfast for two!

VEGGIE BREAKFAST HASH

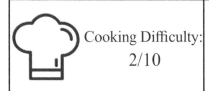 Cooking Difficulty: 2/10

 Cooking Time: 25 minutes

 Servings: 2

INGREDIENTS

- 2 medium potatoes
- 1 large carrot
- 1 red onion
- 2 tablespoons olive oil
- 1/2 teaspoon garlic powder
- 1/2 teaspoon paprika
- salt and pepper to taste
- fresh herbs for serving (such as parsley or cilantro)

DESCRIPTION

STEP 1
Dice the potatoes and carrot into roughly cubes. Halve the red onion and slice it into thin half-moons. Heat olive oil in a skillet over medium heat. Add the diced potatoes and cook, stirring occasionally, until tender, about 10-12 minutes.

STEP 2
Add the diced carrot and sliced red onion to the skillet with the potatoes. Continue cooking, stirring, for an additional 5-7 minutes. Season the veggie hash with garlic powder, paprika, salt, and pepper to taste. Stir well to evenly distribute the spices. Serve.

NUTRITIONAL INFORMATION

200 Calories, 7g Fat, 30g Carbs, 4g Protein

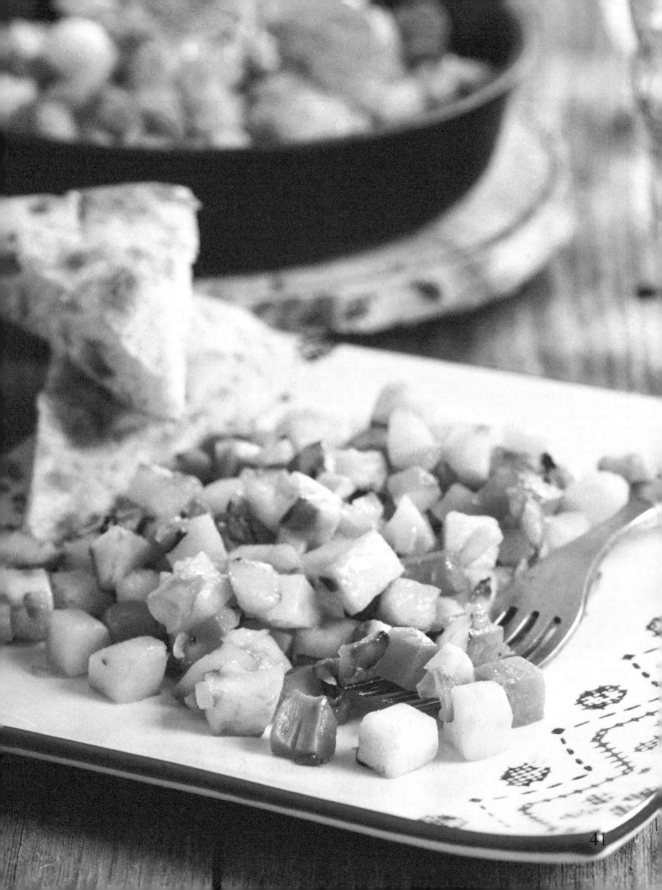

EASY SCOTCH EGGS

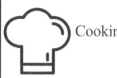 Cooking Difficulty: 3/10

 Cooking Time: 23 minutes

 Servings: 2

INGREDIENTS

- 2 large eggs
- 200g ground turkey or chicken
- 1/2 teaspoon dijon mustard
- salt and pepper to taste
- breadcrumbs for coating
- vegetable oil for frying

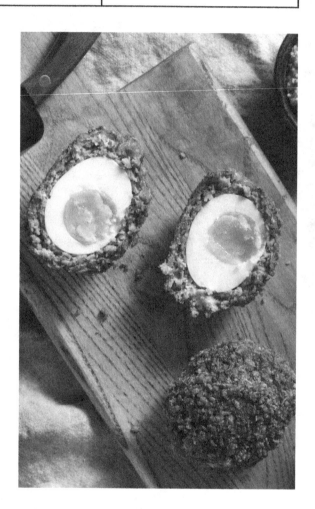

NUTRITIONAL INFORMATION

Calories: 200; Fat: 10 g; Carbs: 5 g; Protein: 15g

STEP 1

Bring a medium saucepan of water to a boil. Carefully lower the eggs into the boiling water and cook for 7-8 minutes for medium-boiled yolks. Then transfer the eggs to cold water to stop the cooking process. Peel the eggs and let them cool.

STEP 2

In a bowl, mix together the ground turkey or chicken with Dijon mustard, salt, and pepper to taste.

STEP 3

Divide the mixture into two portions and shape each portion into a flat circle. Wrap the meat circles around the boiled eggs to form egg «balls.»

STEP 4

Roll the Scotch eggs in breadcrumbs, ensuring even coverage.

STEP 5

Heat vegetable oil in a large skillet over medium heat. Fry the Scotch eggs, turning them occasionally, until golden brown and thoroughly cooked on all sides, about 6-8 minutes.

STEP 6

Serve the Scotch eggs warm or at room temperature.

STEP 7

Enjoy!

TOFU BREAKFAST

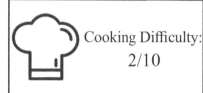 Cooking Difficulty:
2/10

 Cooking Time:
15 minutes

 Servings:
2

INGREDIENTS

- 200g firm tofu, drained and cubed
- 1 onion, sliced
- 1 red bell pepper, sliced
- 1 clove garlic, minced
- 2 tablespoons olive oil
- 1 teaspoon turmeric
- salt and pepper to taste
- fresh herbs for garnish (such as parsley or basil)
- several cherry tomatoes for decoration (optional)

DESCRIPTION

STEP 1
Heat olive oil in a medium skillet over medium heat. Add the sliced onion, red bell pepper, and minced garlic. Sauté, stirring occasionally, for about 5-7 minutes. Add the cubed firm tofu to the skillet with the vegetables. Sprinkle with turmeric and season with salt and pepper to taste. Stir to combine all the ingredients well.

STEP 2
Continue cooking, stirring, for another 5-7 minutes until the tofu is heated through and has a golden color. Serve the tofu breakfast warm, garnished with fresh herbs and decorated with cherry tomatoes if desired.

NUTRITIONAL INFORMATION
200 Calories, 12g Fat, 10g Carbs, 10g Protein

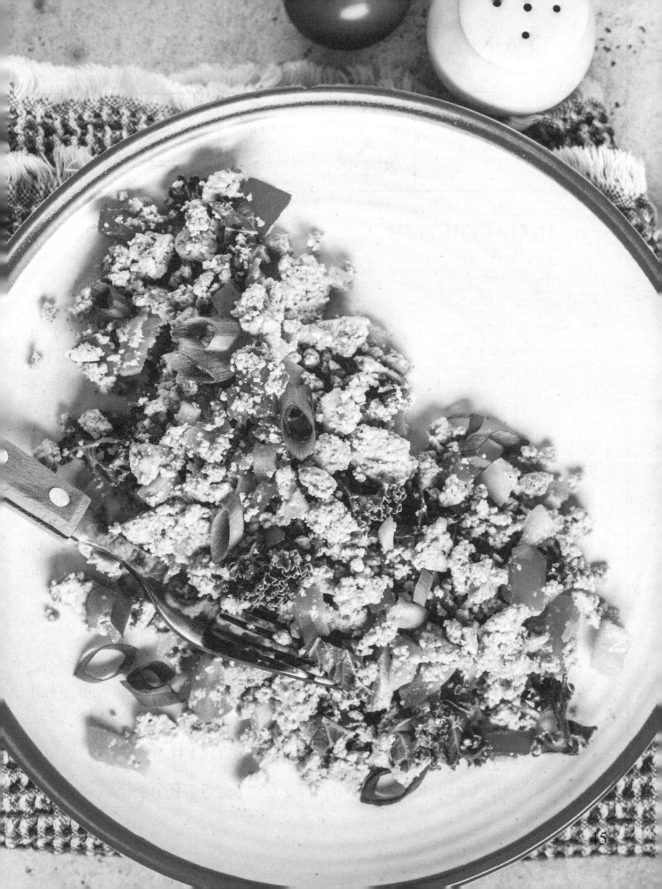

BANANA OAT PANCAKES

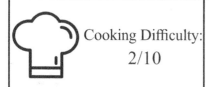 Cooking Difficulty:
2/10

 Cooking Time:
10 minutes

 Servings:
2

INGREDIENTS

- 2 ripe bananas
- 2 eggs
- 1 cup rolled oats
- oil for cooking

DESCRIPTION

STEP 1
In a large bowl, mash the bananas with a fork until smooth. Add the eggs to the mashed bananas and mix well. Stir in the rolled oats until the mixture forms a smooth batter.

STEP 2
Heat a skillet over medium heat and add oil. Pour small amounts of batter onto the skillet to form pancakes. Cook the pancakes until golden brown on both sides. Repeat with the remaining batter.

STEP 3
Serve the pancakes warm with your favorite toppings. Enjoy your meal!

NUTRITIONAL INFORMATION

200 Calories, 3g Fat, 27g Carbs, 5g Protein

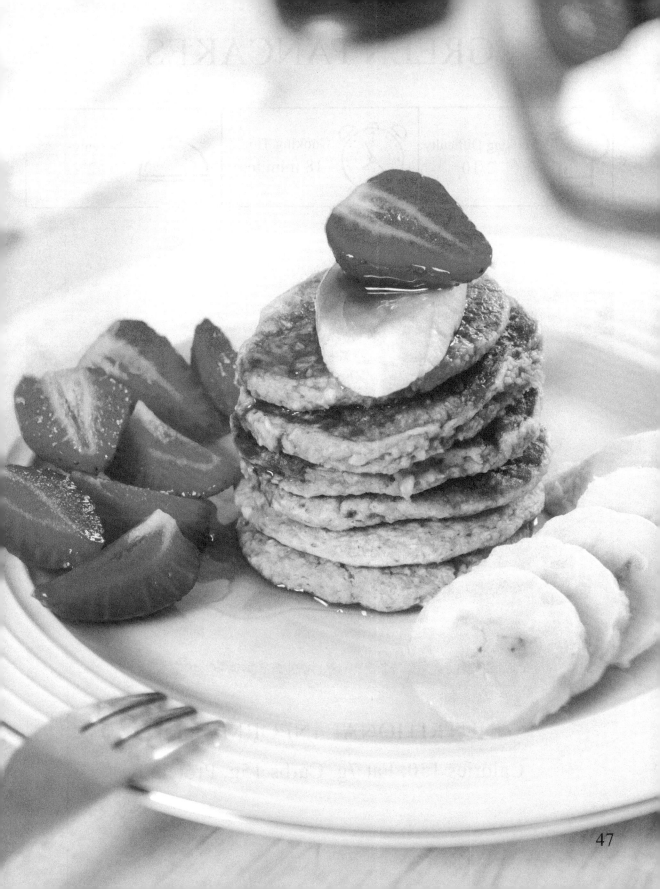

GREEN PANCAKES

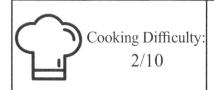 Cooking Difficulty: 2/10	Cooking Time: 18 minutes	Servings: 2

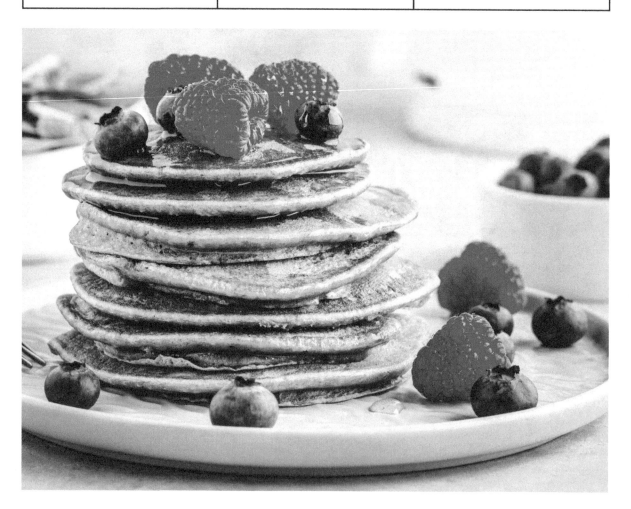

NUTRITIONAL INFORMATION

Calories 150, Fat 7g, Carbs 15g, Protein 6g

INGREDIENTS

- 1 ripe banana
- 2 eggs
- 1 cup chopped spinach
- 1/2 cup rolled oats
- 1 teaspoon baking powder
- pinch of salt
- olive oil for frying

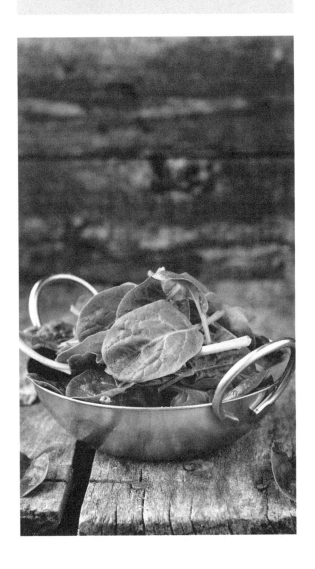

DESCRIPTION

STEP 1
In a blender, combine the ripe banana, eggs, and chopped spinach until smooth. Add the rolled oats, baking powder, and a pinch of salt to the mixture and blend until you have a thick batter.

STEP 2
Heat a skillet or griddle over medium heat. Grease the skillet with olive oil.

STEP 3
Pour a small amount of batter onto the skillet to form pancakes.

STEP 4
Cook until bubbles appear on the surface, then flip and cook until golden brown on the other side.

STEP 5
Repeat with the remaining batter, adding more olive oil as needed. Serve the green pancakes warm with your favorite toppings, such as fresh berries, maple syrup, or Greek yogurt. Enjoy your meal!

SCRAMBLED EGGS WITH ASPARAGUS & GREEN PEAS

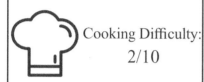 Cooking Difficulty: 2/10	Cooking Time: 10 minutes	Servings: 2

INGREDIENTS

- 4 eggs
- 100g green peas (frozen or fresh)
- 100g asparagus, chopped into pieces
- 100g smoked salmon, sliced
- 2 tbsp olive oil
- salt and pepper to taste
- fresh herbs for garnish (optional)

DESCRIPTION

STEP 1

Beat the eggs in a bowl, season with salt and pepper to taste. Heat olive oil in a skillet over medium heat. Add the asparagus and cook, stirring, for about 3-4 minutes until the asparagus is tender. Add the green peas to the skillet with the asparagus and cook for another 1-2 minutes.

STEP 2

Pour the beaten eggs into the skillet. Cook, stirring, until the eggs are cooked through and scrambled. Divide the scrambled eggs onto plates. Top with slices of smoked salmon and fresh herbs, if desired.

NUTRITIONAL INFORMATION

250 Calories, 15g Fat, 10g Carbs, 20g Protein

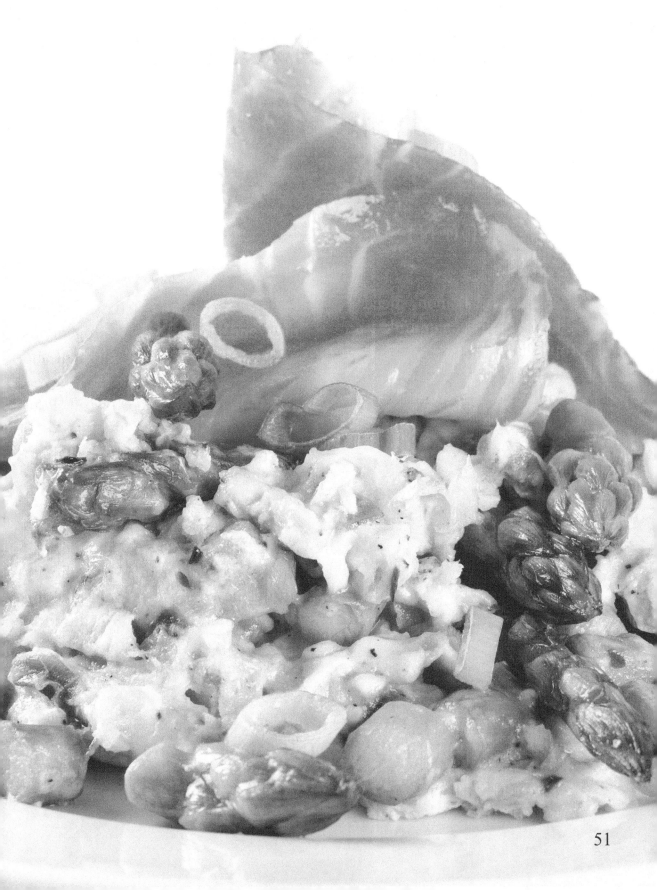

SALMON OMELETTE

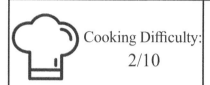 Cooking Difficulty: 2/10

 Cooking Time: 10 minutes

 Servings: 3

INGREDIENTS

- 6 eggs
- 100g smoked salmon, sliced
- 2 tablespoons vegan milk (optional)
- salt and pepper to taste
- 1 tablespoon olive oil

DESCRIPTION

STEP 1

Beat the eggs in a bowl. If desired, add milk and beat until a homogeneous mixture forms. Season with salt and pepper to taste. Heat a skillet over medium heat and add olive oil. Pour half of the beaten eggs into the skillet and spread evenly. Sprinkle half of the sliced smoked salmon over the surface of the eggs.

STEP 2

Cook the omelette, periodically lifting the edges to prevent sticking to the skillet, until the eggs are fully cooked. Repeat the same steps for the second portion of the omelette. Serve!

NUTRITIONAL INFORMATION

200 Calories, 15g Fat, 3g Carbs, 15g Protein

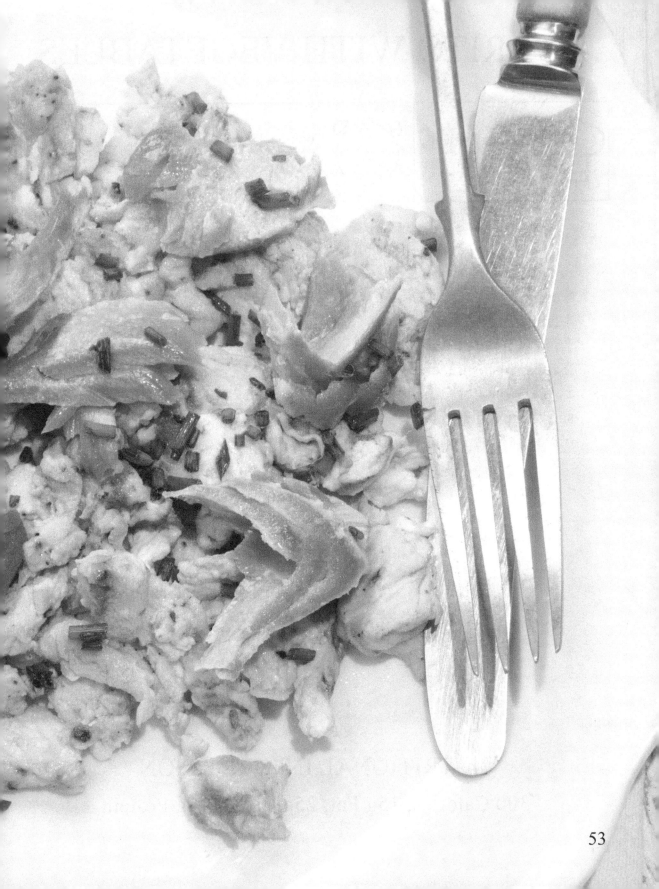

BURRITO WITH VEGETABLES

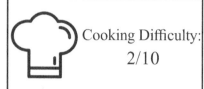 Cooking Difficulty: 2/10

 Cooking Time: 11 minutes

 Servings: 2

INGREDIENTS

- 4 eggs
- 4 large tortillas
- 1 red bell pepper, sliced
- 2 cups fresh spinach
- 2 small tomatoes, diced
- salt and pepper to taste
- olive oil for cooking

DESCRIPTION

STEP 1

In a large skillet, heat a little olive oil over medium heat. Add the red bell pepper to the skillet and cook, until softened, about 5 minutes. Add the fresh spinach to the skillet and cook 2-3 minutes. In a separate bowl, beat the eggs and season with salt and pepper to taste.

STEP 2

Add the beaten eggs to the skillet with the vegetables. Cook, stirring, until the eggs are cooked through. Divide the cooked vegetables and eggs evenly among each tortilla. Roll up the burritos, folding in the sides, to enclose the filling.

NUTRITIONAL INFORMATION

300 Calories, 15g Fat, 25g Carbs, 15g Protein

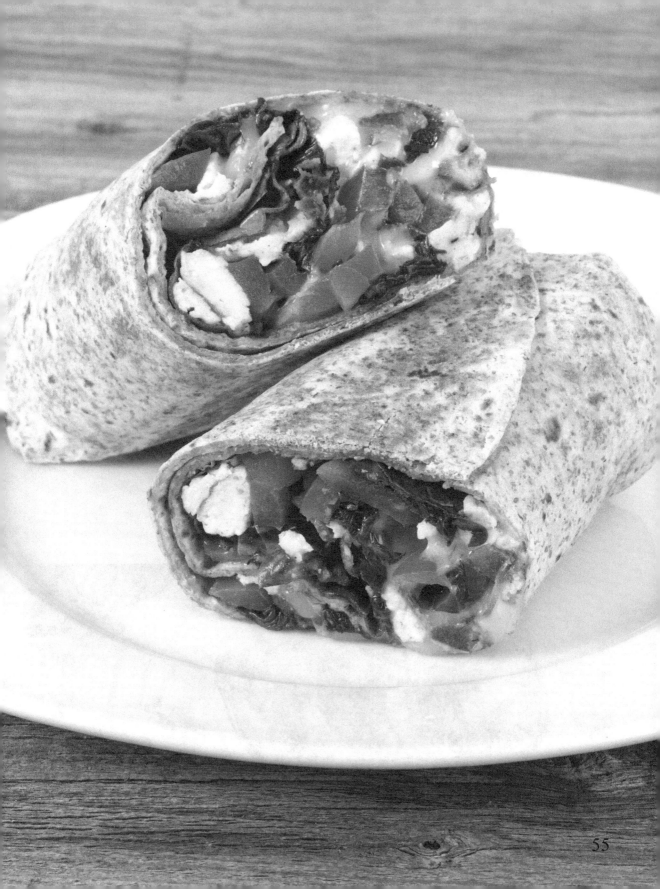

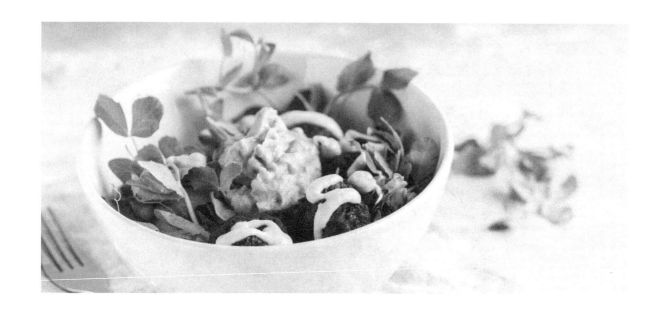

MAIN DISH

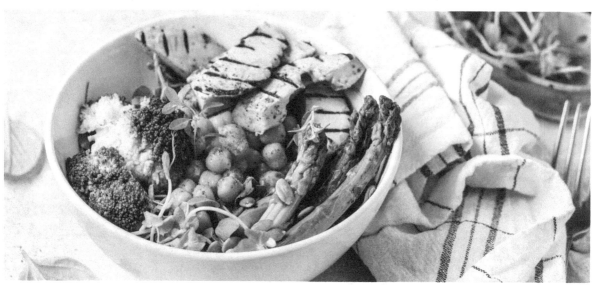

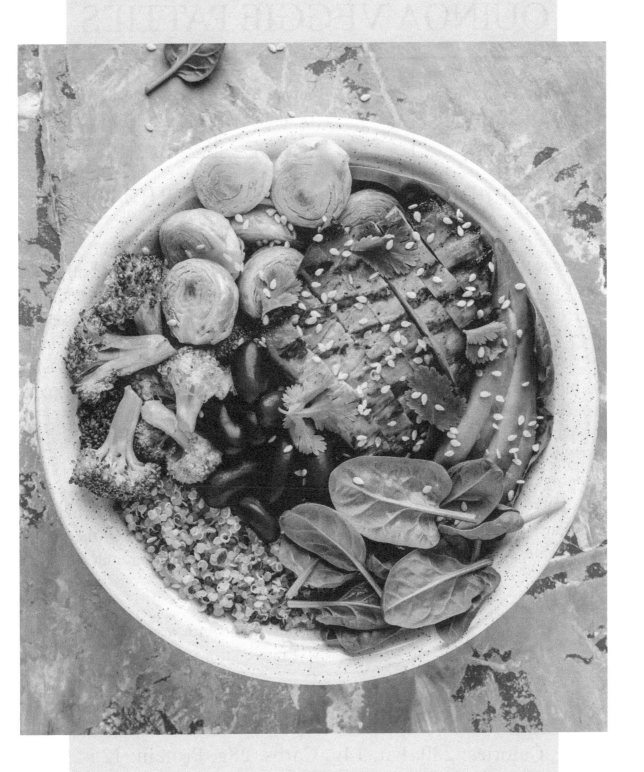

57

QUINOA VEGGIE PATTIES

 Cooking Difficulty: 3/10

 Cooking Time: 18 minutes

 Servings: 2

INGREDIENTS

- 1/2 cup quinoa, rinsed
- 1 cup water
- 1 medium carrot, grated
- 1/2 red onion, finely chopped
- 1 clove garlic, minced
- 1/2 cup cooked chickpeas, mashed
- 2 tablespoons chopped fresh parsley
- salt and pepper to taste
- 1 egg
- 2 tablespoons breadcrumbs or flour
- 2 tablespoons olive oil

DESCRIPTION

STEP 1
Cook quinoa in water until all water is absorbed. In a large bowl, combine cooked quinoa, mashed chickpeas, grated carrot, chopped onion, minced garlic, parsley, salt, pepper, and egg. Add breadcrumbs or flour to help the mixture bind together.

STEP 2
Form the mixture into patties. Heat olive oil in a skillet over medium heat. Cook the patties in the skillet until golden brown on both sides.

STEP 3
Serve hot with your favorite sauce. Enjoy!

NUTRITIONAL INFORMATION

Calories: 280, Fat: 14g, Carbs: 28g, Protein: 12g

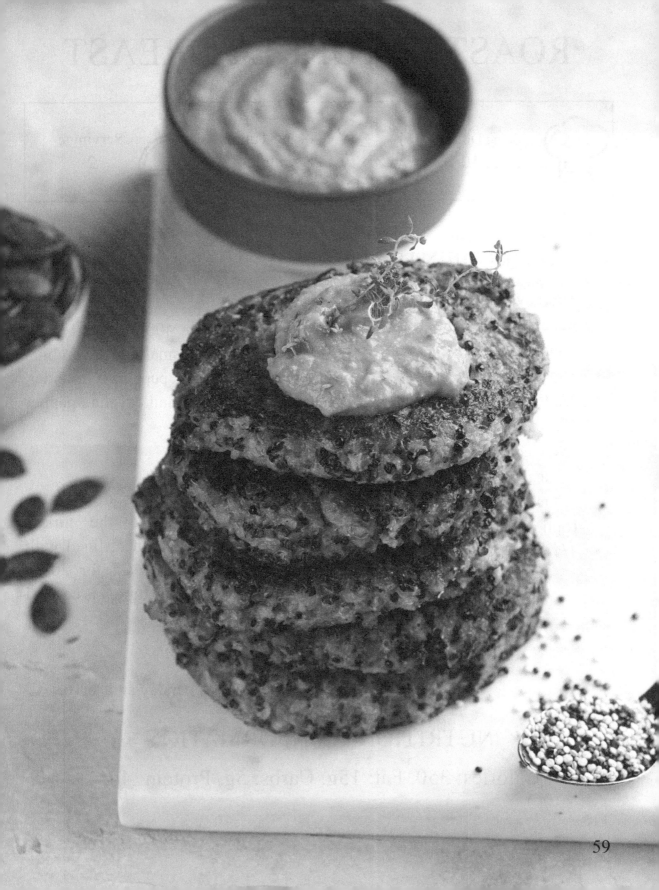

ROASTED TURKEY BREAST

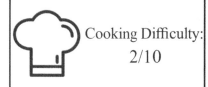 Cooking Difficulty: 2/10	 Cooking Time: 28 minutes	Servings: 2

INGREDIENTS

- 1 turkey breast (about 14 ounces)
- 1 tablespoon olive oil
- 1 teaspoon salt
- 1/2 teaspoon black pepper
- 1/2 teaspoon ground coriander
- 1/4 teaspoon ground cumin
- 1/4 teaspoon paprika
- 1/4 teaspoon cayenne pepper (optional)
- 1/4 cup fresh parsley, chopped

DESCRIPTION

STEP 1
Preheat oven to 400 degrees F (200 degrees C). In a small bowl, combine olive oil, salt, pepper, coriander, cumin, paprika, and cayenne pepper (optional).

STEP 2
Rub the spice mixture all over the turkey breast. Place the turkey breast on a baking sheet lined with parchment paper. Roast for 20-25 minutes, or until the turkey is cooked through.

STEP 3
Sprinkle with parsley and serve.

NUTRITIONAL INFORMATION

Calories: 350, Fat: 15g, Carbs: 5g, Protein: 40g

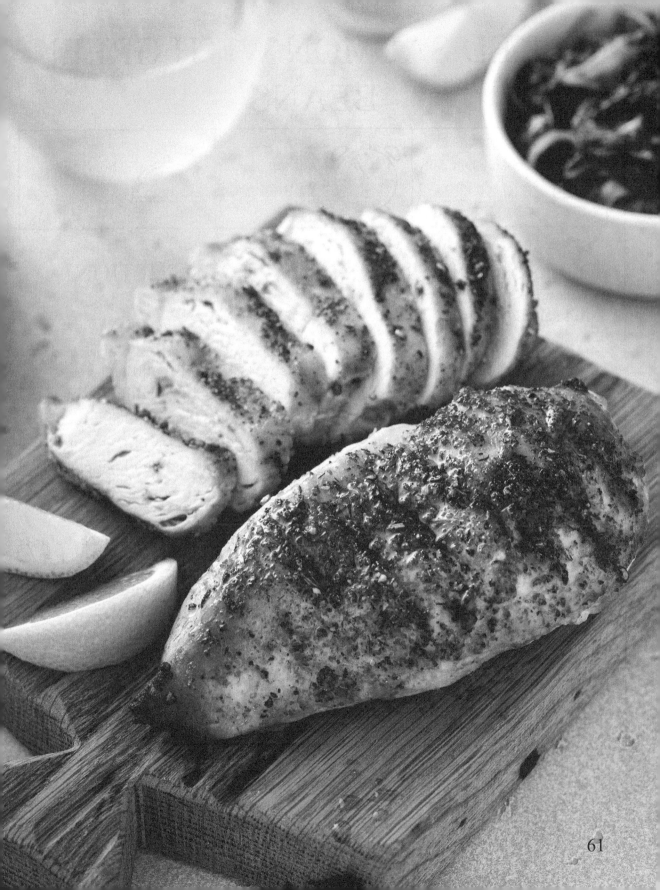

BAKED SALMON WITH GREEN BEANS

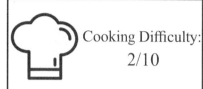 Cooking Difficulty: 2/10	 Cooking Time: 25 minutes	Servings: 4

INGREDIENTS

- 4 salmon fillets (about 5.5 ounces each)
- 14 ounces green beans, trimmed
- 1 tablespoon olive oil
- 1/2 teaspoon salt
- 1/4 teaspoon black pepper
- 1 lemon, sliced
- 1/4 cup fresh parsley, chopped

DESCRIPTION

STEP 1

Preheat oven to 400 degrees F (200 degrees C). Wash and trim the green beans. Blanch in boiling water for 2-3 minutes, then drain and set aside. In a large bowl, toss the green beans with olive oil, salt, and pepper.

STEP 2

Spread the green beans in a baking dish. Place the salmon fillets on top of the green beans. Season the salmon with salt, pepper, and lemon slices. Bake for 15-20 minutes, or until the salmon is cooked through. Garnish with parsley and serve.

NUTRITIONAL INFORMATION

Calories: 400, Fat: 18g, Carbs: 10g, Protein: 30g

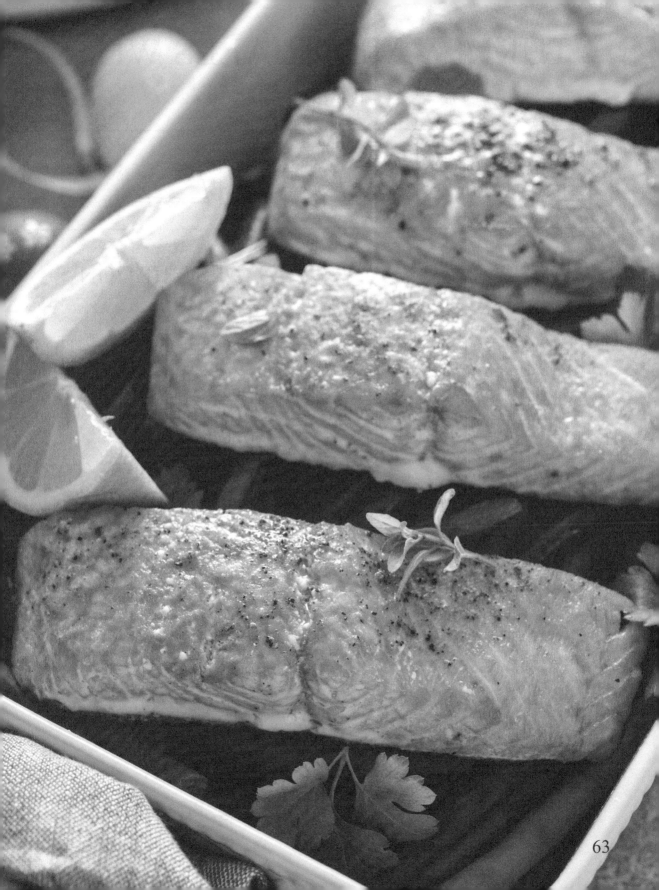

TURKEY MEATBALLS WITH MINT

 Cooking Difficulty: 2/10

 Cooking Time: 27 minutes

 Servings: 4

INGREDIENTS

- 1 pound ground turkey
- 1/2 onion, finely chopped
- 1 clove garlic, minced
- 1/4 cup fresh mint, chopped
- 1/4 cup fresh spinach leaves, chopped
- 1 egg
- 1/4 cup bread crumbs
- 1 tablespoon olive oil
- 1/2 teaspoon salt
- 1/4 teaspoon black pepper
- 1/4 teaspoon nutmeg

DESCRIPTION

STEP 1
Preheat oven to 350 degrees F (175 degrees C). In a large bowl, combine turkey, onion, garlic, mint, spinach, egg, bread crumbs, olive oil, salt, pepper, and nutmeg.

STEP 2
Shape the mixture into 1-inch meatballs. Place meatballs on a baking sheet lined with parchment paper. Bake for 20-25 minutes, or until meatballs are browned and cooked through.

STEP 3
Serve with your favorite sauce, such as tomato sauce, yogurt sauce, or pesto.

NUTRITIONAL INFORMATION

Calories: 350, Fat: 15g, Carbs: 10g, Protein: 35g

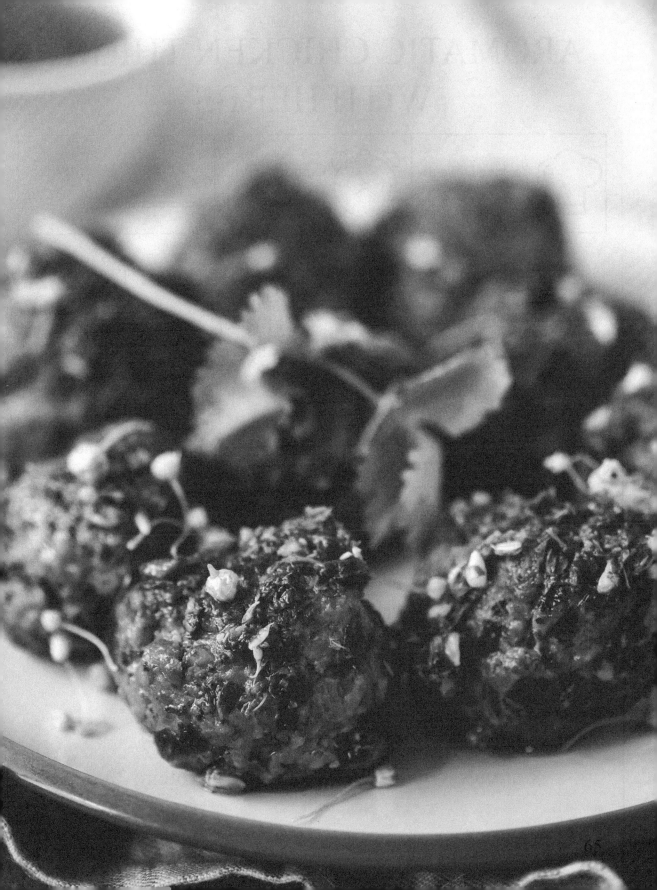

AROMATIC CHICKEN THIGHS WITH HERBS

Cooking Difficulty: 2/10	Cooking Time: 45 minutes	Servings: 4

INGREDIENTS

- 4 chicken thighs (about 1 pound)
- 2 tablespoons olive oil
- 1 teaspoon salt
- 1/2 teaspoon black pepper
- 1/2 teaspoon paprika
- 1/4 teaspoon garlic powder
- 1/4 teaspoon onion powder
- 1/4 teaspoon smoked paprika
- 1/4 teaspoon ground cumin
- 1/8 teaspoon cayenne pepper (optional)
- 1/4 cup fresh parsley, chopped

DESCRIPTION

STEP 1
Preheat oven to 400 degrees F (200 degrees C). In a small bowl, combine olive oil, salt, pepper, paprika, garlic powder, onion powder, smoked paprika, cumin, and cayenne pepper (optional). Rub the spice mixture all over the chicken thighs.

STEP 2
Place the chicken thighs on a baking sheet lined with parchment paper. Roast for 35-45 minutes, or until the chicken is cooked through and the juices run clear. Sprinkle with parsley and serve.

NUTRITIONAL INFORMATION

Calories: 400, Fat: 25g, Carbs: 5g, Protein: 30g

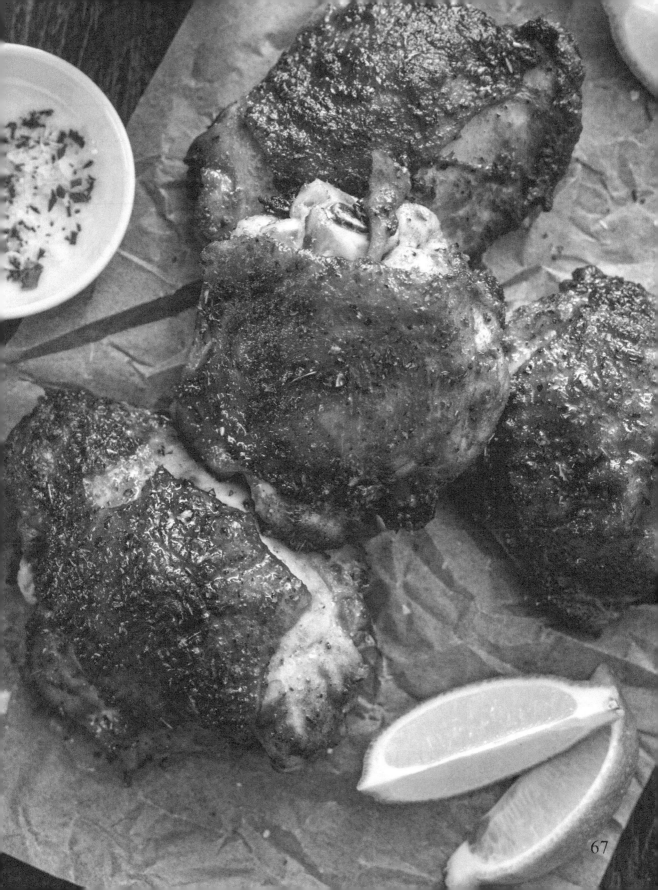

TOMATO BASIL SOUP

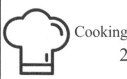 Cooking Difficulty: 2/10	 Cooking Time: 27 minutes	Servings: 2

INGREDIENTS

- 1 (14.5-ounce) can diced tomatoes, undrained
- 1 onion, chopped
- 1 clove garlic, minced
- 1 bell pepper, chopped
- 2 tablespoons olive oil
- 2 cups vegetable broth
- 1/2 teaspoon dried oregano
- 1/4 teaspoon black pepper
- salt to taste
- 2 fresh basil leaves, thinly sliced

DESCRIPTION

STEP 1
In a large pot, heat the olive oil over medium heat. Add the onion, garlic, and bell pepper and cook until softened, about 5 minutes.

STEP 2
Stir in the diced tomatoes, vegetable broth, oregano, black pepper, and salt. Bring to a boil, then reduce heat and simmer for 20 minutes. Remove from heat and let cool slightly.

STEP 3
Using an immersion blender or regular blender, blend the soup until smooth and creamy. Stir in the fresh basil. Serve hot.

NUTRITIONAL INFORMATION

Calories: 200, Fat: 10g, Carbs: 25g, Protein: 10g

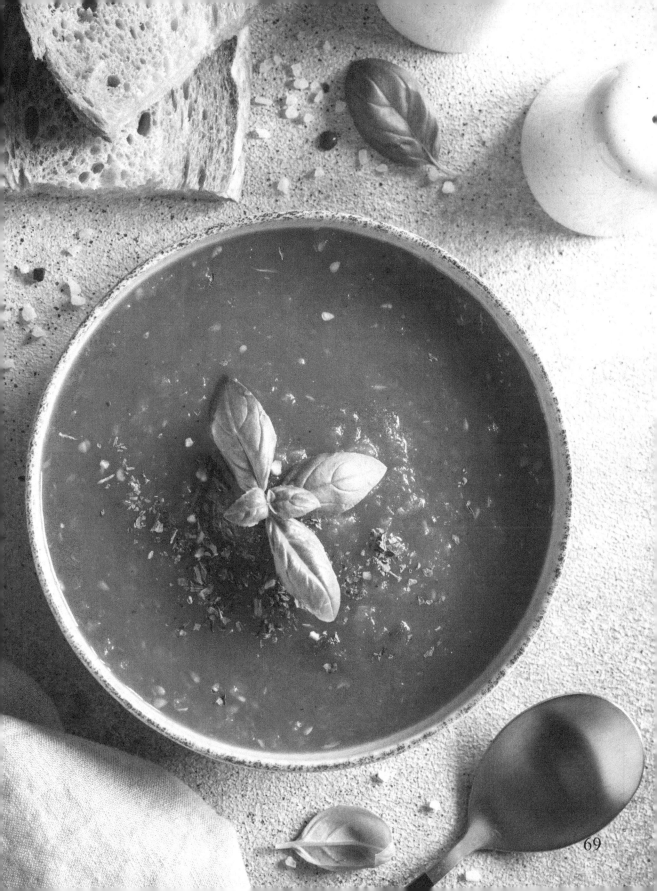

VEGGIE ROAST

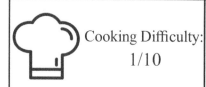 Cooking Difficulty: 1/10

 Cooking Time: 30 minutes

 Servings: 2

INGREDIENTS

- 1 cup broccoli florets
- 1 cup cauliflower florets
- 2 tablespoons olive oil
- 1/2 teaspoon salt
- 1/4 teaspoon black pepper
- 1/4 teaspoon paprika

DESCRIPTION

STEP 1
Preheat oven to 400 degrees F (200 degrees C). In a large bowl, toss broccoli, cauliflower, olive oil, salt, pepper, and paprika.

STEP 2
Spread vegetables in a single layer on a baking sheet lined with parchment paper.

STEP 3
Roast for 20-25 minutes, or until vegetables are tender and slightly crispy.

NUTRITIONAL INFORMATION

Calories: 150, Fat: 10g, Carbs: 10g, Protein: 5g

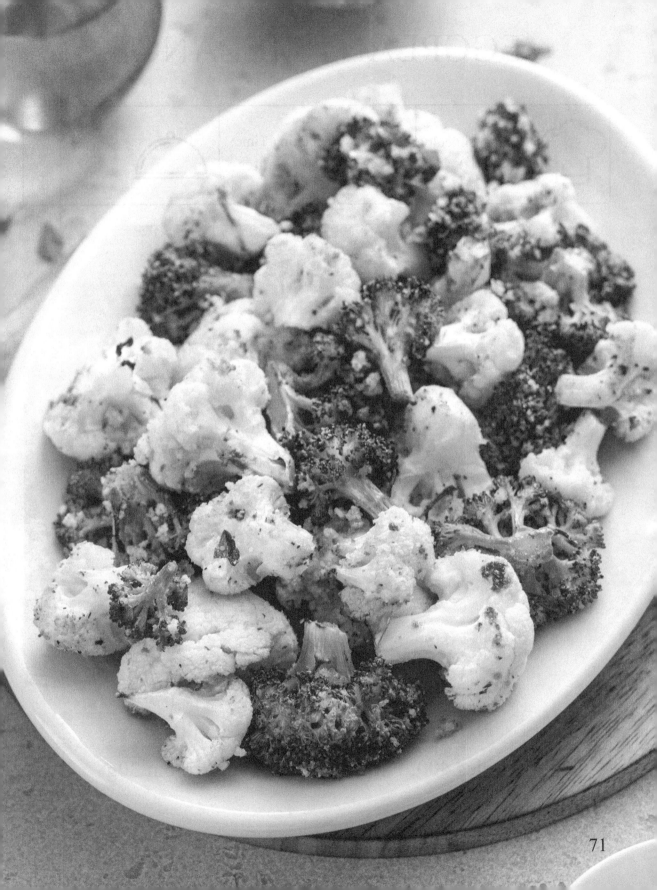

EGGPLANT MELANGE

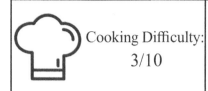 Cooking Difficulty: 3/10	Cooking Time: 34 minutes	Servings: 2

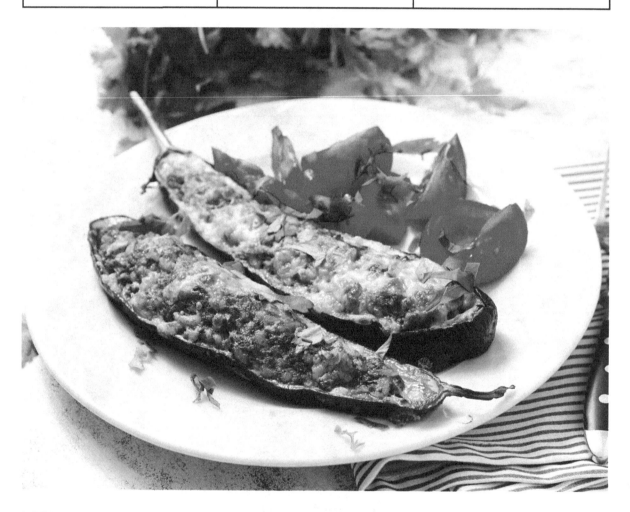

NUTRITIONAL INFORMATION

Calories 400, Fat 20g, Carbs 25g, Protein 30g

INGREDIENTS

- 1 large eggplant
- 1 pound ground chicken
- 1 cup chopped mushrooms
- 1/2 onion, chopped
- 1 clove garlic, minced
- 1 tablespoon olive oil
- 1/2 teaspoon dried oregano
- 1/4 teaspoon salt
- 1/4 teaspoon black pepper
- 1/4 cup shredded vegan mozzarella cheese (optional)

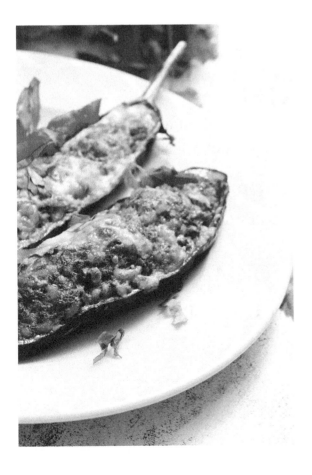

DESCRIPTION

STEP 1

Preheat oven to 375 degrees F (190 degrees C). Cut the eggplant in half lengthwise and scoop out the flesh, leaving a 1/2-inch shell. Chop the eggplant flesh and set aside.

STEP 2

In a large skillet, heat the olive oil over medium heat. Add the onion and cook until softened, about 5 minutes. Add the garlic and cook for 30 seconds more, until fragrant.

STEP 3

Add the ground chicken and cook, breaking it up with a spoon, until browned. Drain off any excess grease. Stir in the chopped mushrooms, oregano, salt, and pepper. Cook for 5 minutes more, or until the mushrooms are tender.

STEP 4

Stir in the reserved chopped eggplant flesh. Divide the chicken mixture among the eggplant halves.Sprinkle with mozzarella cheese. Bake for 20-25 minutes, or until the eggplants are tender.

SPINACH AND BROCCOLI SOUP

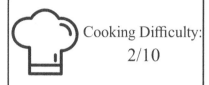 Cooking Difficulty: 2/10

 Cooking Time: 27 minutes

 Servings: 2

INGREDIENTS

- 1 tablespoon olive oil
- 1 onion, diced
- 2 cloves garlic, minced
- 1 cup broccoli florets
- 1 cup frozen spinach
- 3 cups vegetable broth
- ⅓ cup unsweetened coconut milk (optional)
- salt and pepper to taste

DESCRIPTION

STEP 1
Sauté onion and garlic, add broccoli and spinach, cook until softened.

STEP 2
Pour in vegetable broth, bring to a boil, simmer 15 minutes.

STEP 3
Blend until smooth, add coconut milk (optional), salt, and pepper.

STEP 4
Heat through, serve hot.

NUTRITIONAL INFORMATION

Calories: 200, Fat: 10g, Carbs: 10g, Protein: 5g

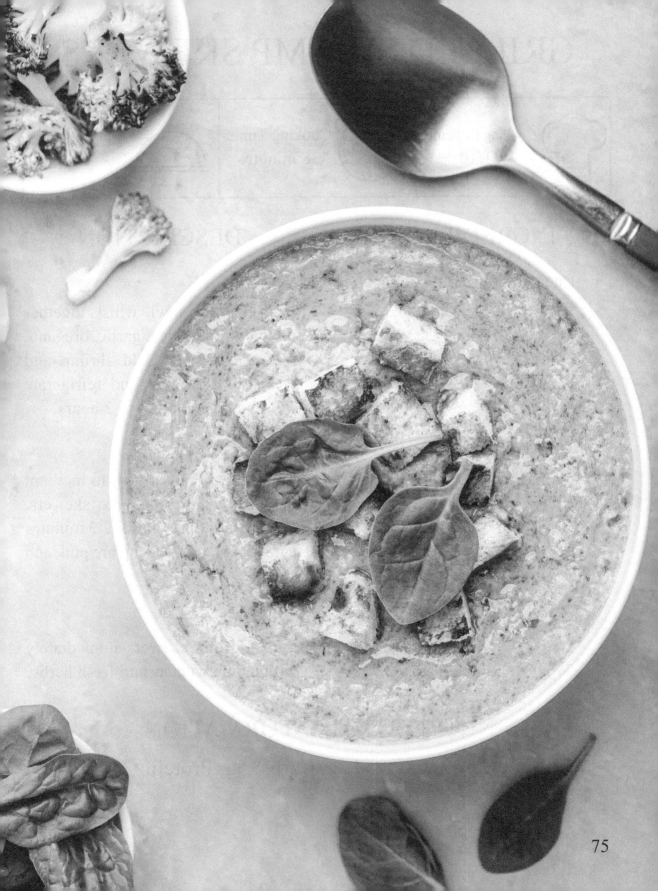

GRILLED SHRIMP SKEWERS

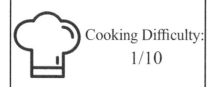 Cooking Difficulty:
1/10

 Cooking Time:
38 minutes

 Servings:
2

INGREDIENTS

- 1 pound large shrimp, tails on and unpeeled
- ¼ cup olive oil
- 2 tablespoons lime juice
- 1 tablespoon minced garlic
- 1 teaspoon dried oregano
- ½ teaspoon salt
- ¼ teaspoon black pepper
- ¼ cup chopped fresh parsley (optional)

DESCRIPTION

STEP 1
In a medium bowl, whisk together olive oil, lime juice, garlic, oregano, salt, and pepper. Add shrimp and toss to coat. Cover and refrigerate for 30 minutes, or up to 2 hours.

STEP 2
Preheat grill pan or grill to medium heat. Thread shrimp onto skewers, leaving tails on. Grill for 2-3 minutes per side, or until shrimp are pink and opaque.

STEP 3
Serve shrimp skewers immediately with lemon wedges and fresh herbs.

NUTRITIONAL INFORMATION
Calories: 350, Fat: 15g, Carbs: 5g, Protein: 35g

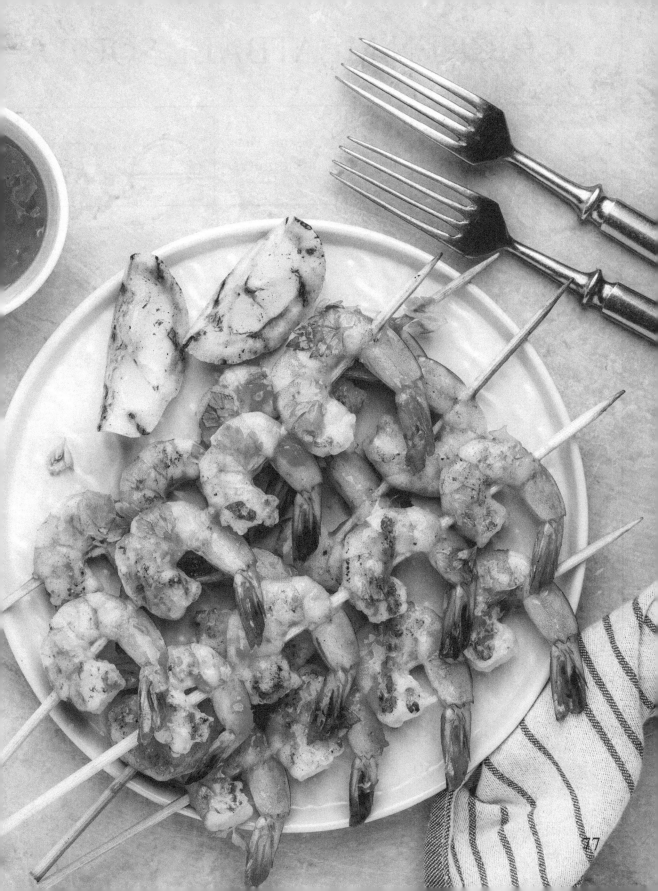

CHICKEN MEATBALL SOUP

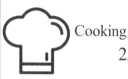 Cooking Difficulty: 2/10

 Cooking Time: 40 minutes

 Servings: 3

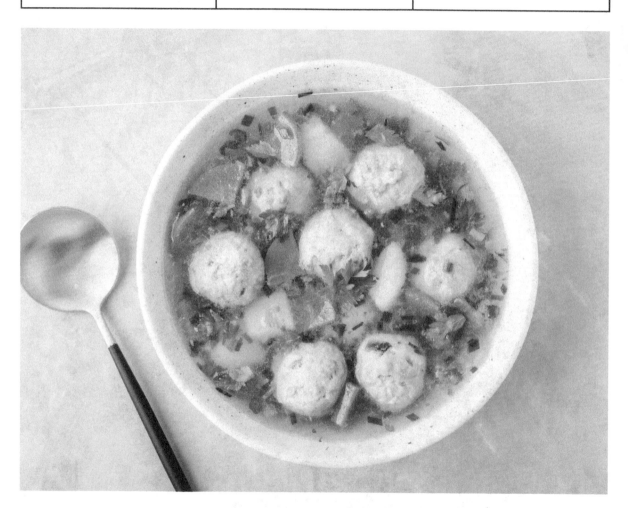

NUTRITIONAL INFORMATION

Calories 350, Fat 15g, Carbs 30g, Protein 25g

INGREDIENTS

for the meatballs:
- 1 pound ground chicken
- 1 onion, finely chopped
- 1 egg
- 2 tablespoons breadcrumbs
- 1 tablespoon milk
- salt and pepper to taste

for the soup:
- 8 cups vegetable broth
- 3 potatoes, diced
- 2 carrots, diced
- 1 bay leaf
- 3-4 black peppercorns
- salt and pepper to taste
- fresh herbs for garnish (optional)

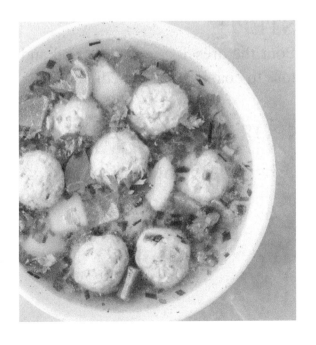

DESCRIPTION

STEP 1
In a bowl, combine the ground chicken, onion, egg, breadcrumbs, milk, salt, and pepper. Mix well until the mixture is evenly distributed. Shape the mixture into small meatballs.

STEP 2
In a large pot, bring the vegetable broth to a boil. Add the potatoes, carrots, bay leaf, and black peppercorns. Cook for 10-15 minutes, or until the vegetables are tender.

STEP 3
Gently drop the meatballs into the simmering soup and cook for an additional 10-15 minutes, or until the meatballs are cooked through and float to the top. Season with salt and pepper to taste.

STEP 4
Ladle the soup into bowls and garnish with fresh herbs, if desired.

CARROT AND RED CABBAGE SALAD

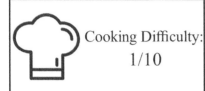 Cooking Difficulty: 1/10	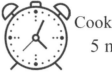 Cooking Time: 5 minutes	Servings: 2

INGREDIENTS

- 2 cups shredded carrots
- 2 cups shredded red cabbage
- 1/4 cup chopped fresh parsley
- 2 tablespoons olive oil
- 1 tablespoon lemon juice
- 1 tablespoon honey
- salt and pepper to taste

DESCRIPTION

STEP 1
In a large bowl, combine the shredded carrots, red cabbage, and parsley.

STEP 2
In a small bowl, whisk together the olive oil, lemon juice, honey, salt, and pepper.

STEP 3
Pour the dressing over the salad and toss to coat. Serve immediately.

NUTRITIONAL INFORMATION

Calories: 200, Fat: 10g, Carbs: 20g, Protein: 2g

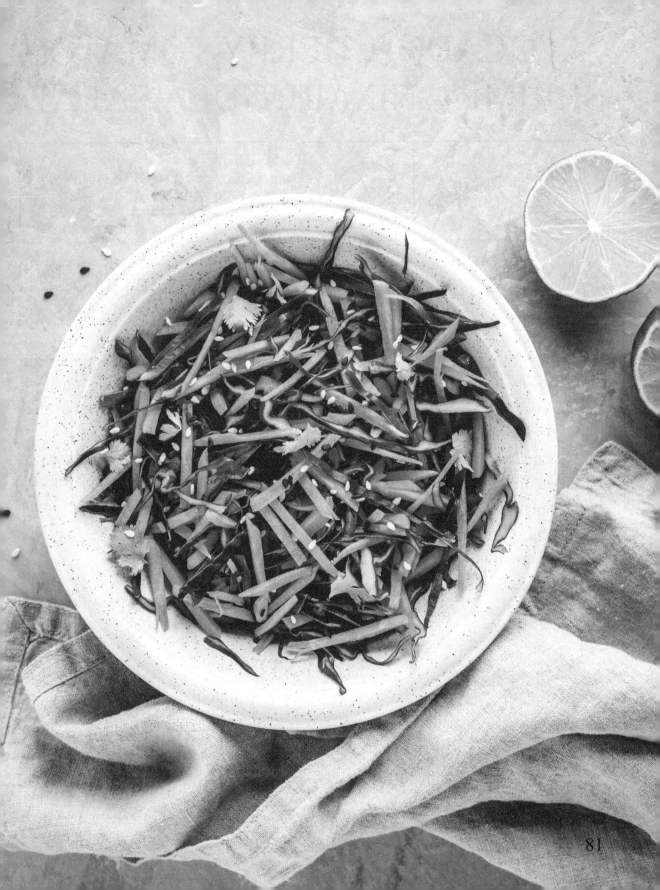

AVOCADO, CHERRY TOMATO, SHRIMP, AND ARUGULA SALAD

 Cooking Difficulty: 1/10

 Cooking Time: 5 minutes

 Servings: 2

INGREDIENTS

for the salad:
- 4 cups baby arugula
- 1 ripe avocado, halved, pitted, and sliced
- 1 cup cherry tomatoes, halved
- 12 cooked and peeled shrimp

for the vinaigrette:
- 2 tablespoons olive oil
- 1 tablespoon lemon juice
- 1 teaspoon dijon mustard
- 1/2 teaspoon dried oregano
- salt and pepper to taste

DESCRIPTION

STEP 1
In a small bowl, whisk together the olive oil, lemon juice, Dijon mustard, oregano, salt, and pepper. Set aside.

STEP 2
In a large bowl, combine the arugula, avocado, cherry tomatoes, and shrimp.

STEP 3
Drizzle the vinaigrette over the salad and toss gently to coat.

STEP 4
Serve immediately and enjoy!

NUTRITIONAL INFORMATION

Calories: 200, Fat: 15g, Carbs: 17g, Protein: 24g

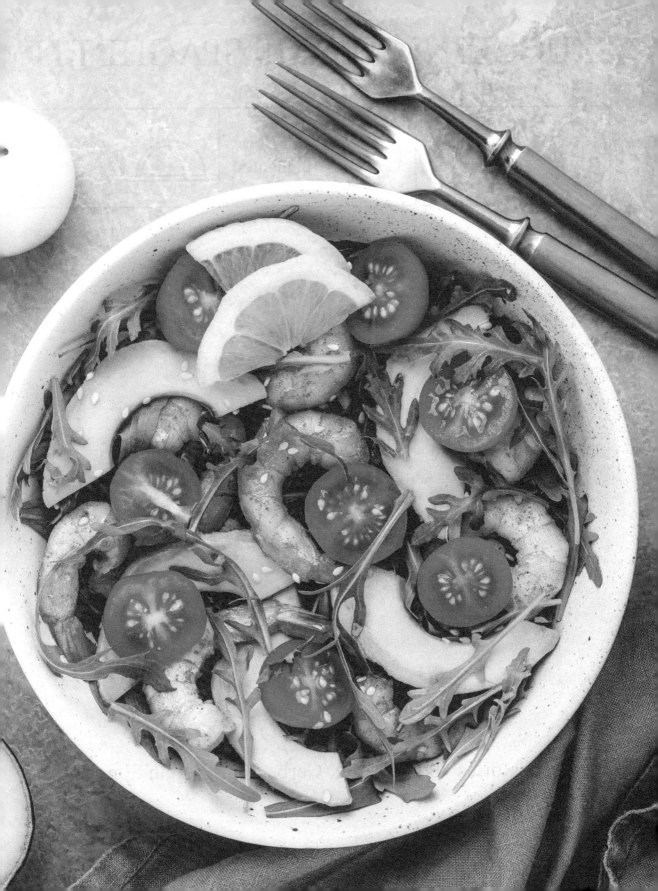

ZUCCHINI SHRIMP SPAGHETTI

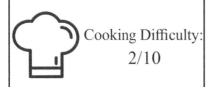 Cooking Difficulty: 2/10

 Cooking Time: 13 minutes

 Servings: 2

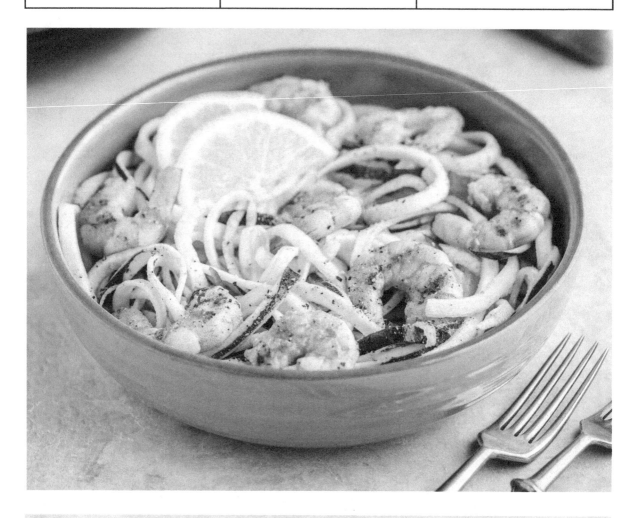

NUTRITIONAL INFORMATION

Calories 400, Fat 15g, Carbs 30g, Protein 30g

INGREDIENTS

- for the pasta:
- 8 ounces zucchini, spiralized or thinly sliced
- 1 tablespoon olive oil
- 2 cloves garlic, minced
- 1/2 teaspoon salt
- 1/4 teaspoon black pepper
- for the shrimp:
- 1 pound shrimp, peeled and deveined
- 1 tablespoon olive oil
- 2 cloves garlic, minced
- 1/4 cup white wine (optional)
- 1/4 cup lemon juice
- 1/4 teaspoon salt
- 1/4 teaspoon black pepper
- 1/4 cup chopped fresh parsley

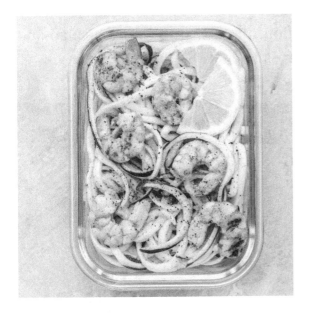

DESCRIPTION

STEP 1
Heat the olive oil in a large skillet over medium heat. Add the garlic and cook for 30 seconds, or until fragrant. Add the zucchini, salt, and pepper and cook for 5-7 minutes, or until tender-crisp.

STEP 2
In a separate skillet, heat the olive oil over medium heat. Add the garlic and cook for 30 seconds, or until fragrant. Add the shrimp and cook for 2-3 minutes per side, or until pink and cooked through.

STEP 3
Add the cooked shrimp to the skillet with the zucchini. Stir in the white wine, lemon juice, salt, and pepper. Bring to a simmer and cook for 1-2 minutes, or until the sauce is heated through.

STEP 4
Garnish with parsley, if desired.

TUNA SALAD WITH SPINACH

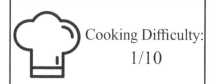 Cooking Difficulty: 1/10

 Cooking Time: 2 minutes

 Servings: 2

INGREDIENTS

- 1 (5-ounce) can tuna in olive oil, drained and flaked
- 4 cups baby spinach
- 1/2 cup sun-dried tomatoes, sliced
- 1/2 cup cooked white beans, drained and rinsed
- 1/4 cup whole olives, pitted
- 1/4 cup red onion, thinly sliced
- 2 tablespoons olive oil
- 1 tablespoon lemon juice
- 1/2 teaspoon salt
- 1/4 teaspoon black pepper

DESCRIPTION

STEP 1
In a large bowl, combine the tuna, spinach, sun-dried tomatoes, white beans, olives, and red onion.

STEP 2
In a small bowl, whisk together the olive oil, lemon juice, salt, and pepper.

STEP 3
Pour the dressing over the salad and toss to coat. Serve immediately.

NUTRITIONAL INFORMATION

Calories: 350, Fat: 15g, Carbs: 30g, Protein: 25g

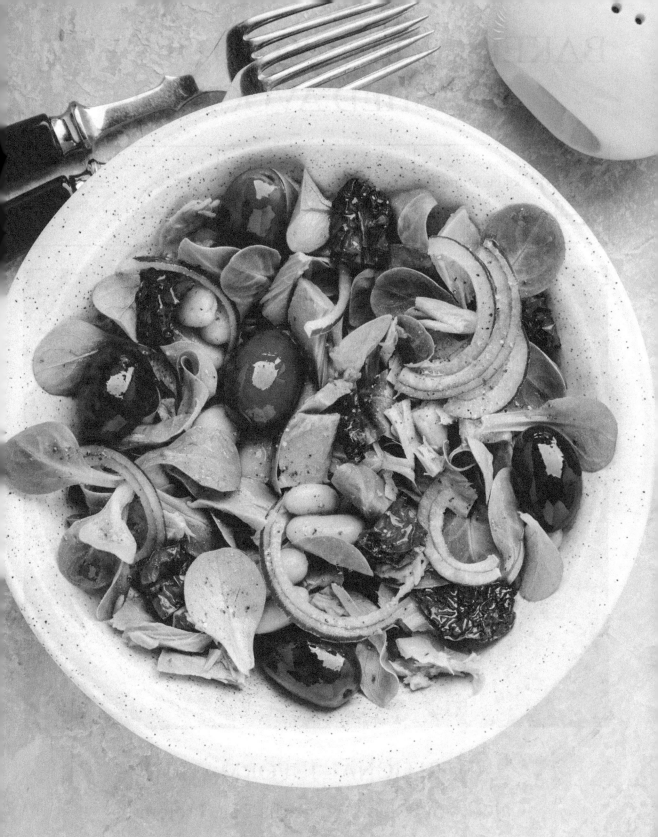

BAKED SWEET POTATOES WITH MASHED AVOCADO

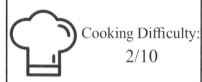 Cooking Difficulty: 2/10

 Cooking Time: 10 minutes

 Servings: 4

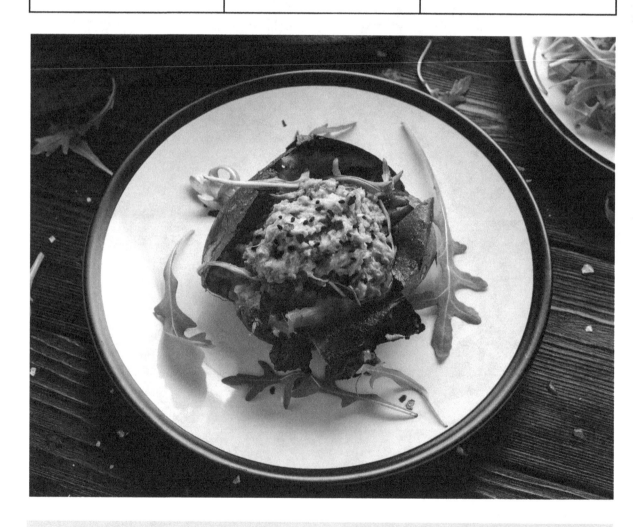

NUTRITIONAL INFORMATION

Calories 300, Fat 10g, Carbs 27g, Protein 9g

INGREDIENTS

- 4 large sweet potatoes
- 2 tablespoons olive oil
- salt and pepper to taste
- 2 avocados, peeled and mashed
- juice of 1 lemon
- 1/2 teaspoon chili powder (or to taste)

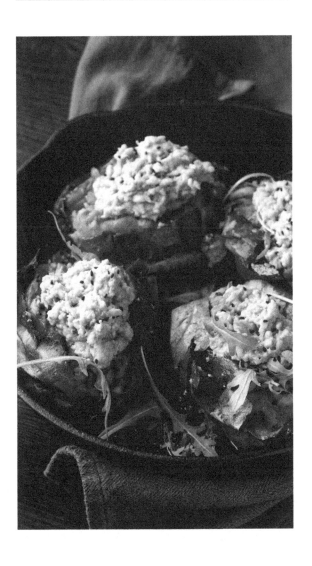

DESCRIPTION

STEP 1
Preheat your air fryer to 200°C (400°F). Wash the sweet potatoes and pierce them all over with a fork. Place them on a baking sheet, drizzle with olive oil, and season with salt and pepper to taste.

STEP 2
Air fry the sweet potatoes for 45-50 minutes, or until they are soft and golden.

STEP 3
While the sweet potatoes are cooking, prepare the mashed avocado. In a bowl, combine mashed avocados with lemon juice and chili powder. Mix well to combine.

STEP 4
Once the sweet potatoes are done, remove them from the air fryer and let them cool slightly. Then, slice each sweet potato lengthwise down the middle, without cutting all the way through.

STEP 5
Fill each sweet potato with the mashed avocado mixture. Enjoy!

CHICKPEA SALAD WITH CHERRY TOMATOES

Cooking Difficulty: 1/10	Cooking Time: 2 minutes	Servings: 2

INGREDIENTS

- 1 cup cooked chickpeas
- 1/2 cup cherry tomatoes, halved
- 1/4 cup red onion, thinly sliced
- 5 cups mixed salad greens (such as arugula, spinach, romaine)
- 1/4 cup crumbled feta cheese (optional)

for the dressing:
- 2 tablespoons olive oil
- 1 tablespoon lemon juice
- 1 teaspoon honey
- 1/2 teaspoon oregano
- salt and pepper to taste

DESCRIPTION

STEP 1
In a large bowl, combine the chickpeas, cherry tomatoes, red onion, and salad greens.

STEP 2
In a small bowl, whisk together the olive oil, lemon juice, honey, oregano, salt, and pepper.

STEP 3
Pour the dressing over the salad and toss gently to coat.

STEP 4
Add the feta cheese (if using) and serve immediately.

NUTRITIONAL INFORMATION

Calories: 210, Fat: 5g, Carbs: 9g, Protein: 15g

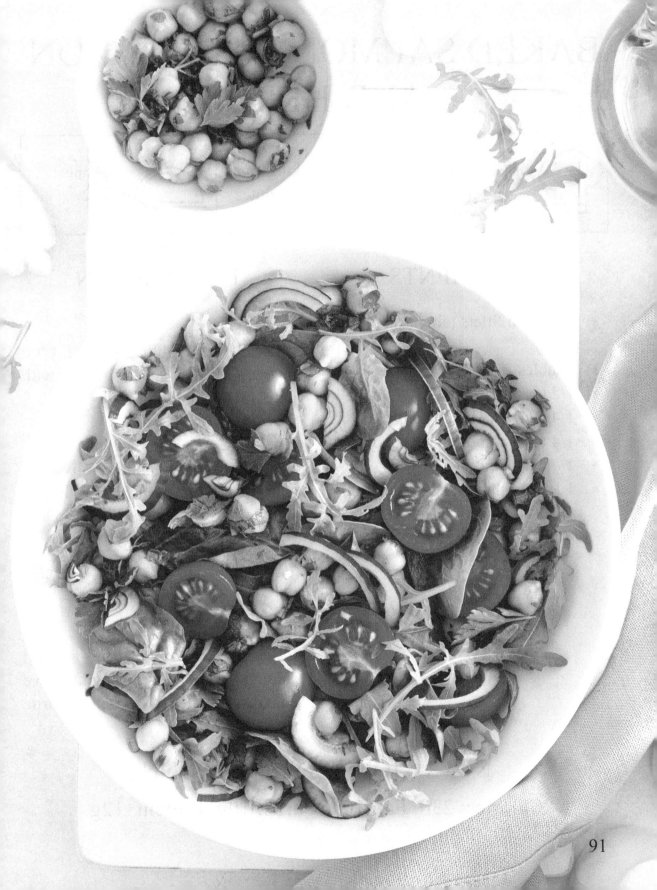

BAKED SALMON WITH LEMON AND HERBS

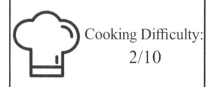 Cooking Difficulty: 2/10

 Cooking Time: 25 minutes

 Servings: 2

INGREDIENTS

- 2 salmon fillets (about 6 ounces each)
- 1 tablespoon olive oil
- 1/2 teaspoon salt
- 1/4 teaspoon black pepper
- 1/4 teaspoon dried oregano
- 1/4 teaspoon dried thyme
- 1 lemon, thinly sliced (optional)

DESCRIPTION

STEP 1
Preheat oven to 400 degrees F (200 degrees C). Line a baking sheet with parchment paper.

STEP 2
In a small bowl, combine olive oil, salt, pepper, oregano, and thyme. Place salmon fillets on the prepared baking sheet and spread the spice mixture evenly over them. Top with lemon slices, if using.

STEP 3
Bake for 15-20 minutes, or until salmon is cooked through. Serve baked salmon with your favorite vegetables.

NUTRITIONAL INFORMATION

Calories: 230, Fat: 10g, Carbs: 10g, Protein: 12g

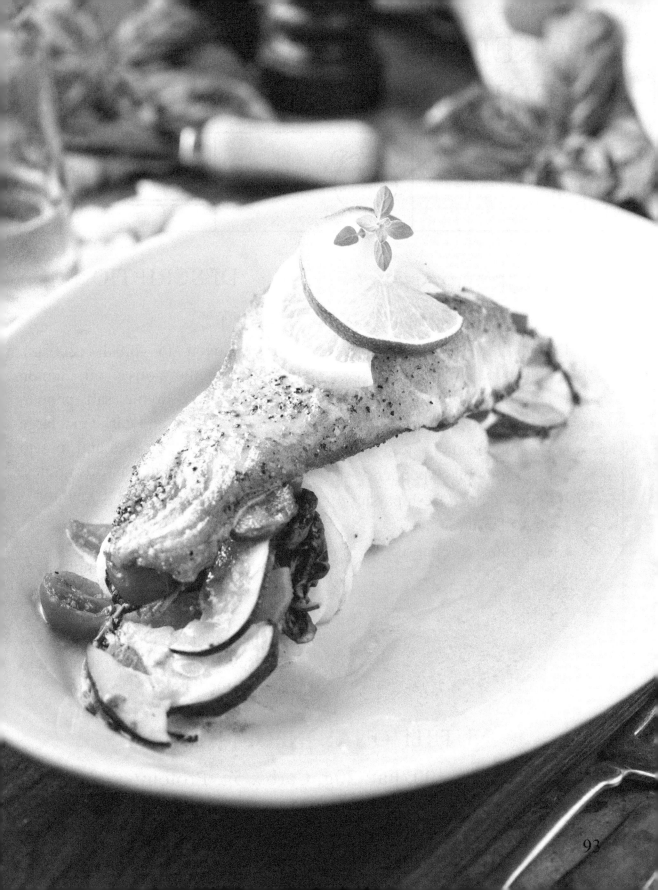

BAKED CHICKEN LEGS WITH A MEDITERRANEAN MARINADE

 Cooking Difficulty: 2/10

 Cooking Time: 57 minutes

 Servings: 2

INGREDIENTS

- 4 bone-in, skin-on chicken legs
- 1/4 cup olive oil
- 2 tablespoons lemon juice
- 1 tablespoon dried oregano
- 1 teaspoon dried thyme
- 1/2 teaspoon salt
- 1/4 teaspoon black pepper
- 1/4 cup chopped fresh parsley
- 2 cloves garlic, minced
- 1 teaspoon sweet paprika

DESCRIPTION

STEP 1
Preheat oven to 400°F (200°C). Whisk together olive oil, lemon juice, oregano, thyme, salt, pepper, paprika, parsley, and garlic in a large bowl. Add chicken legs and toss to coat. Marinate for at least 30 minutes, or up to 4 hours in the refrigerator.

STEP 2
Arrange chicken legs in a single layer in a baking dish. Pour marinade over chicken. Bake for 40-50 minutes, or until cooked through and skin is crispy. Garnish with parsley and serve immediately.

NUTRITIONAL INFORMATION

Calories: 400, Fat: 20g, Carbs: 5g, Protein: 35g

94

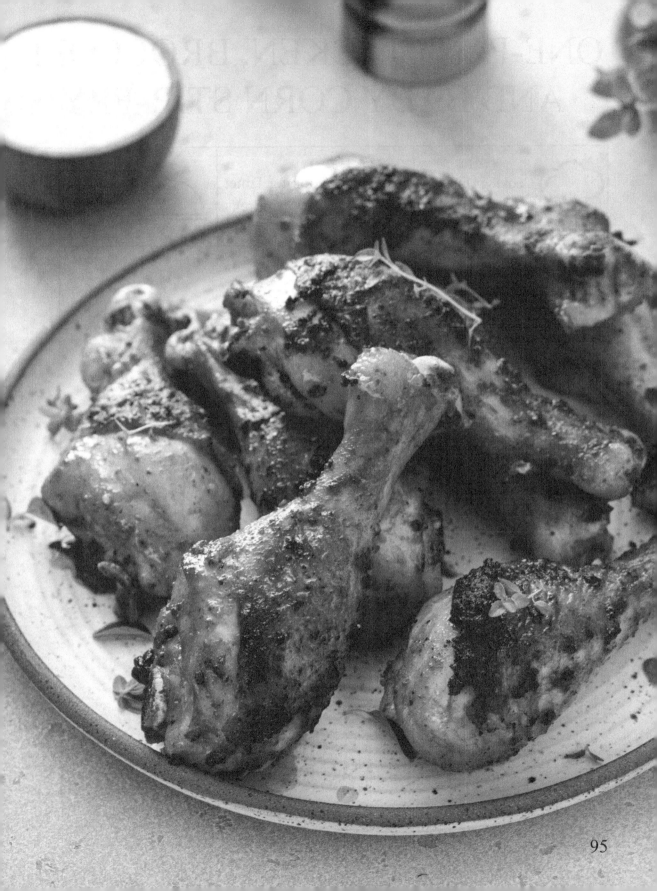

ONE-PAN CHICKEN, BROCCOLI, AND BABY CORN STIR-FRY

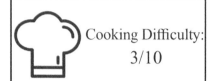 Cooking Difficulty: 3/10

 Cooking Time: 10 minutes

 Servings: 4

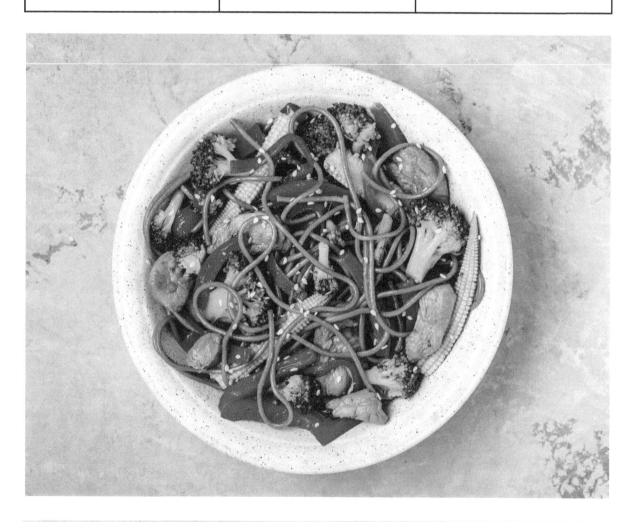

NUTRITIONAL INFORMATION

Calories 400, Fat 15g, Carbs 30g, Protein 30g

INGREDIENTS

- 1 pound boneless, skinless chicken breasts, cut into bite-sized pieces
- 1 tablespoon olive oil
- 1 red bell pepper, thinly sliced
- 1 head of broccoli, cut into florets
- 1 cup baby corn, trimmed
- 1/4 cup soy sauce
- 1 tablespoon honey
- 1 tablespoon rice vinegar
- 1 teaspoon sesame oil
- 1/2 teaspoon minced ginger
- 1/4 teaspoon garlic powder
- salt and pepper to taste

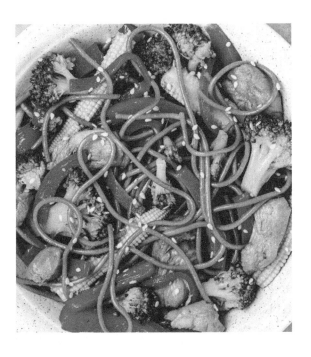

DESCRIPTION

STEP 1
Heat the olive oil in a large skillet or wok over medium-high heat.

STEP 2
Add the chicken and cook until browned on all sides and cooked through, about 5 minutes. Remove the chicken from the pan and set aside.

STEP 3
Add the bell pepper, broccoli, and baby corn to the pan and cook until tender-crisp, about 5 minutes.

STEP 4
In a small bowl, whisk together the soy sauce, honey, rice vinegar, sesame oil, ginger, and garlic powder. Pour the sauce over the vegetables and toss to coat.

STEP 5
Return the chicken to the pan and stir to combine. Season with salt and pepper to taste. Serve immediately over noodles. Enjoy!

ANCHOVY SALAD WITH EGG AND CHERRY TOMATOES

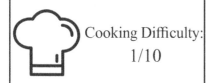 Cooking Difficulty: 1/10

 Cooking Time: 5 minutes

 Servings: 2

INGREDIENTS

- 1 oz anchovies in oil
- 1 oz kalamata olives
- 2.5 oz cherry tomatoes
- 1/4 red onion, thinly sliced
- 2.5 oz spinach
- 1 hard-boiled egg, sliced
- 1 tablespoon olive oil
- 1 tablespoon lemon juice
- salt and pepper to taste

DESCRIPTION

STEP 1
Rinse the anchovies under cold running water to remove excess salt. Chop them finely.

STEP 2
Slice the kalamata olives into rings. Halve the cherry tomatoes. In a large bowl, combine spinach, cherry tomatoes, red onion, and olives. Add the chopped anchovies and sliced egg.

STEP 3
In a small bowl, whisk together olive oil, lemon juice, salt, and pepper. Dress the salad with the prepared mixture and toss gently.

NUTRITIONAL INFORMATION
Calories: 280, Fat: 8g, Carbs: 8g, Protein: 4g

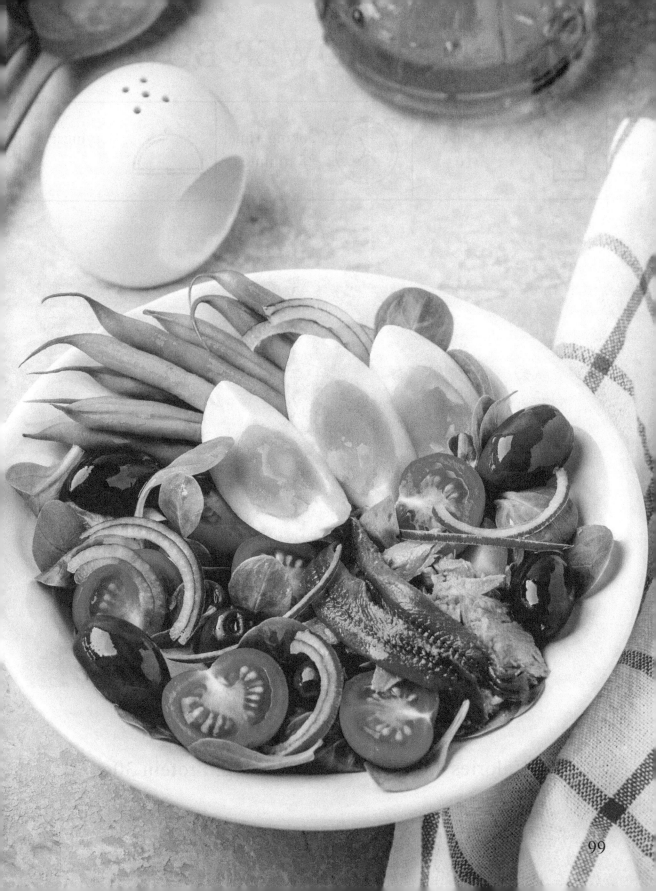

SHRIMP POWER BOWL

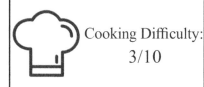 Cooking Difficulty: 3/10	Cooking Time: 25 minutes	Servings: 2

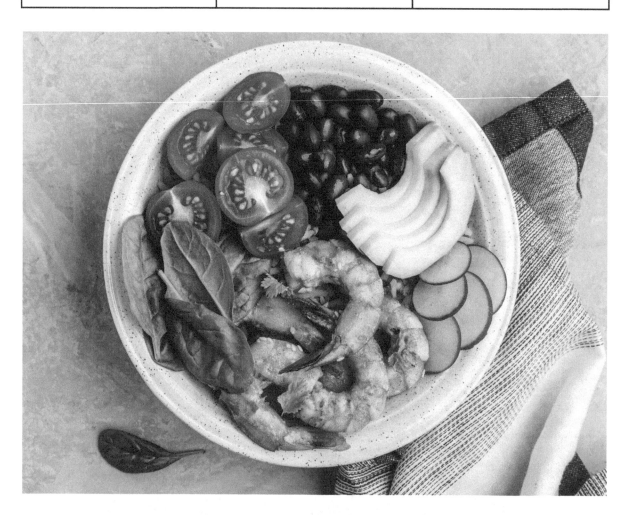

NUTRITIONAL INFORMATION

Calories 450, Fat 18g, Carbs 45g, Protein 30g

INGREDIENTS

for the rice:
- 1/2 cup (100 g) brown rice or quinoa, cooked according to package directions

for the shrimp:
- 1 pound (450 g) shrimp, peeled and deveined
- 1 tablespoon olive oil
- 1/2 teaspoon garlic powder
- 1/4 teaspoon salt
- 1/4 teaspoon black pepper

for the toppings:
- 1 can (15 ounces) red kidney beans, drained and rinsed
- 1 avocado, sliced
- 5 radishes, thinly sliced
- 10 cherry tomatoes, halved
- 2 tablespoons chopped cilantro

for the dressing:
- 1/4 cup olive oil
- 2 tablespoons lime juice
- 1 tablespoon honey
- 1 teaspoon dijon mustard
- 1/2 teaspoon salt
- 1/4 teaspoon black pepper

DESCRIPTION

STEP 1

Cook the rice or quinoa according to package directions.

STEP 2

In a medium bowl, combine the shrimp, olive oil, garlic powder, salt, and pepper. Let marinate for 5 minutes.

STEP 3

Heat a large skillet over medium-high heat. Add the shrimp and cook until pink and cooked through, about 2-3 minutes per side.

STEP 4

Divide the rice or quinoa evenly among two bowls. Top with the shrimp, red kidney beans, avocado, radishes, cherry tomatoes, and cilantro.

STEP 5

In a small bowl, whisk together the olive oil, lime juice, honey, Dijon mustard, salt, and pepper. Drizzle the dressing over the bowls and serve immediately.

LEMON HERB BAKED CHICKEN

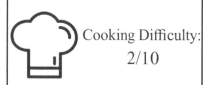 Cooking Difficulty: 2/10

 Cooking Time: 57 minutes

 Servings: 4

INGREDIENTS

- 4 boneless, skinless chicken breasts (about 3 lbs)
- 2 tablespoons olive oil
- 1 tablespoon lemon juice
- 1 teaspoon dried oregano
- 1/2 teaspoon dried thyme
- 1/4 teaspoon garlic powder
- 1/4 teaspoon paprika
- salt and freshly ground black pepper to taste
- 1 pound (450 g) green beans, trimmed and cut into bite-sized pieces
- 1 lemon, thinly sliced

DESCRIPTION

STEP 1
Preheat your oven to 400°F (200°C). In a small bowl, whisk together olive oil, lemon juice, oregano, thyme, garlic powder, paprika, salt, and pepper.

STEP 2
Place chicken breasts in a baking dish. Pour the marinade over the chicken, ensuring they're evenly coated. Arrange the green beans around the chicken breasts. Top with lemon slices.

STEP 3
Bake for 30-35 minutes, or until the chicken is cooked through. Let the chicken rest for a few minutes before serving.

NUTRITIONAL INFORMATION

Calories: 300, Fat: 12g, Carbs: 15g, Protein: 35g

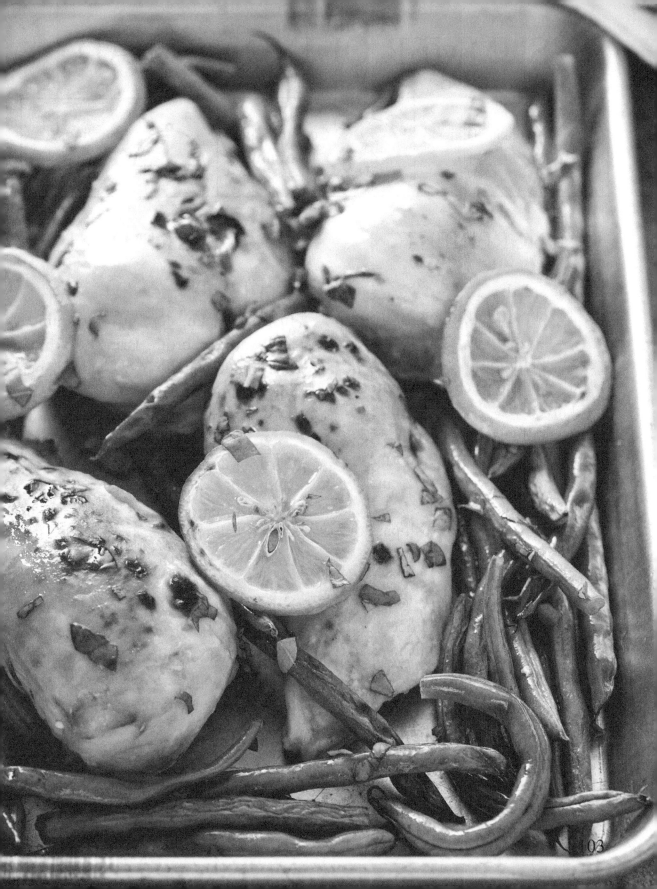

SUMMER QUINOA SALAD

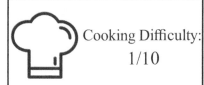 Cooking Difficulty: 1/10	 Cooking Time: 18 minutes	Servings: 2

INGREDIENTS

for the salad:
- 1/2 cup (100 g) quinoa, rinsed
- 1 cup (240 ml) water or vegetable broth
- 1 cup (150 g) cherry tomatoes, halved
- 1 small zucchini, diced
- 1/2 cup (75 g) frozen corn kernels, thawed (or 1/2 cup fresh corn kernels)
- 1/4 cup (chopped fresh parsley or cilantro)

for the dressing:
- 2 tablespoons olive oil
- 1 tablespoon lemon juice
- 1/2 teaspoon dijon mustard
- salt and freshly ground black pepper to taste

DESCRIPTION

STEP 1
In a saucepan, combine the quinoa and water or broth. Bring to a boil, then reduce heat, cover, and simmer for 15 minutes, or until the quinoa is cooked through and fluffy.

STEP 2
While the quinoa cools, halve the cherry tomatoes, dice the zucchini, and fresh corn kernels. Chop the parsley or cilantro.

STEP 3
In a small bowl, whisk together the olive oil, lemon juice, Dijon mustard, salt, and pepper. Pour the dressing over the salad and toss gently to coat.

NUTRITIONAL INFORMATION

Calories: 250, Fat: 5g, Carbs: 7g, Protein: 11g

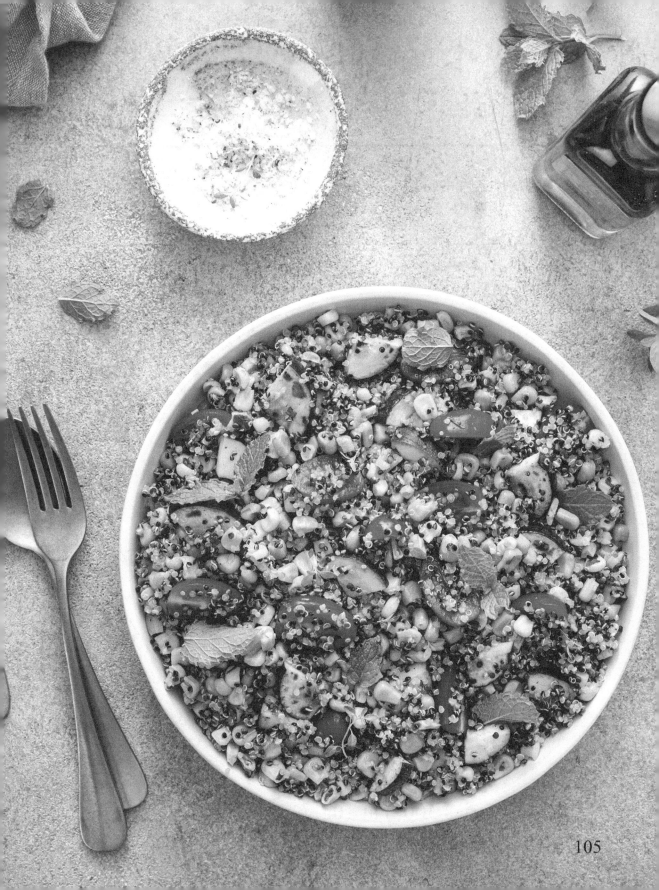

VEGGIE TOSTADAS WITH GUACAMOLE

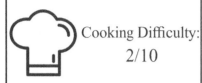 Cooking Difficulty: 2/10	Cooking Time: 15 minutes	Servings: 2

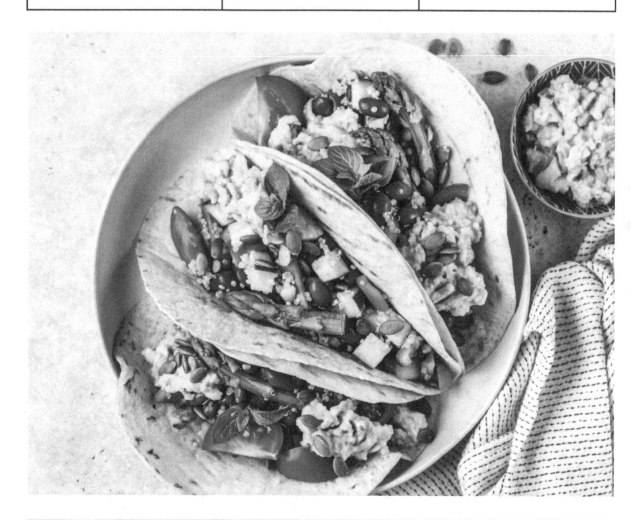

NUTRITIONAL INFORMATION

Calories 300, Fat 10g, Carbs 27g, Protein 9g

INGREDIENTS

- 2 tortillas (wheat or corn)
- 1/2 red bell pepper, sliced into half rings
- 1/2 green bell pepper, sliced into half rings
- 1/2 red onion, sliced
- 1/2 teaspoon cumin
- 1/2 teaspoon chili powder
- salt and pepper to taste
- 1 tablespoon olive oil
- 1 large tomato, diced
- 1 avocado
- 1/2 lime, juice
- 1 clove garlic, minced
- fresh cilantro or parsley for serving
- 1/2 can of canned beans (e.g., black or red beans), rinsed and drained

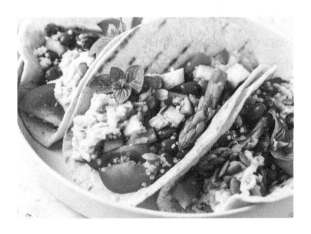

DESCRIPTION

STEP 1
Preheat the air fryer to 200°C (390°F). In a large bowl, mix the red bell pepper, green bell pepper, red onion, cumin, chili powder, salt, pepper, and olive oil.

STEP 2
Spread the vegetable mixture evenly on the tortillas and carefully transfer them to the air fryer.

STEP 3
Cook the tostadas for 8-10 minutes or until the vegetables are tender and golden brown.

STEP 4
While the tostadas are cooking, prepare the guacamole. In a bowl, mash the avocado, add lime juice, minced garlic, salt, and pepper to taste. Mix well until smooth.

STEP 5
Once the tostadas are ready, top each one with diced tomatoes, beans, and a generous amount of guacamole. Serve the hot veggie tostadas with lime wedges.

ZUCCHINI FRITTERS

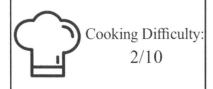 Cooking Difficulty: 2/10	 Cooking Time: 20 minutes	Servings: 2

INGREDIENTS

- 1 medium zucchini, grated
- 1 egg
- 2 tablespoons flour
- 1 tablespoon chopped fresh herbs (dill, parsley, cilantro)
- 1 clove garlic, minced
- 1/4 teaspoon salt
- 1/4 teaspoon black pepper
- vegetable oil for frying

DESCRIPTION

STEP 1
Grate the zucchini and squeeze out excess moisture.

STEP 2
In a bowl, combine zucchini, egg, flour, herbs, garlic, salt, and pepper.

STEP 3
Heat oil in a skillet over medium heat. Drop spoonfuls of batter into the skillet and cook for 2-3 minutes per side, or until golden brown.

STEP 4
Serve warm with your favorite dipping sauce.

NUTRITIONAL INFORMATION

Calories: 150, Fat: 6g, Carbs: 15g, Protein: 5g

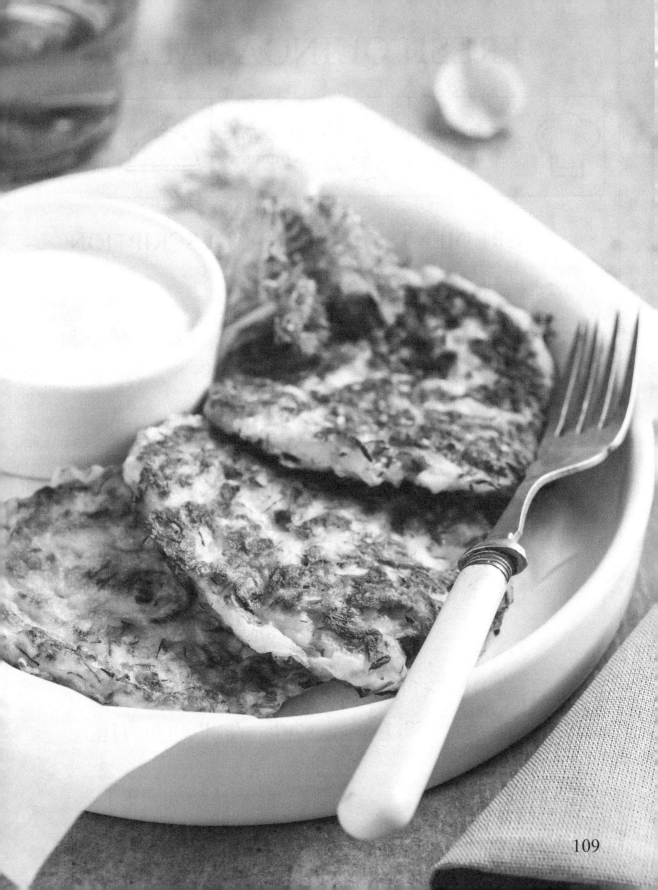

FRESH QUINOA SALAD

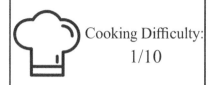 Cooking Difficulty: 1/10

 Cooking Time: 18 minutes

 Servings: 2

INGREDIENTS

- 1/2 cup (100 g) quinoa, rinsed
- 1 cup (240 ml) water or vegetable broth
- 1 cup (50 g) baby spinach
- 1 cup (150 g) cherry tomatoes, halved
- 1/4 cup (30 g) red onion, thinly sliced
- 2 tablespoons olive oil
- 1 tablespoon lemon juice
- salt and freshly ground black pepper to taste

DESCRIPTION

STEP 1
Cook quinoa according to package instructions (about 15 minutes). Let cool slightly.

STEP 2
Combine quinoa, spinach, tomatoes, and red onion in a large bowl. In a small bowl, whisk together olive oil, lemon juice, salt, and pepper.

STEP 3
Pour the dressing over the salad and toss to coat. Serve immediately or refrigerate for up to 2 days.

NUTRITIONAL INFORMATION

Calories: 250, Fat: 5g, Carbs: 7g, Protein: 11g

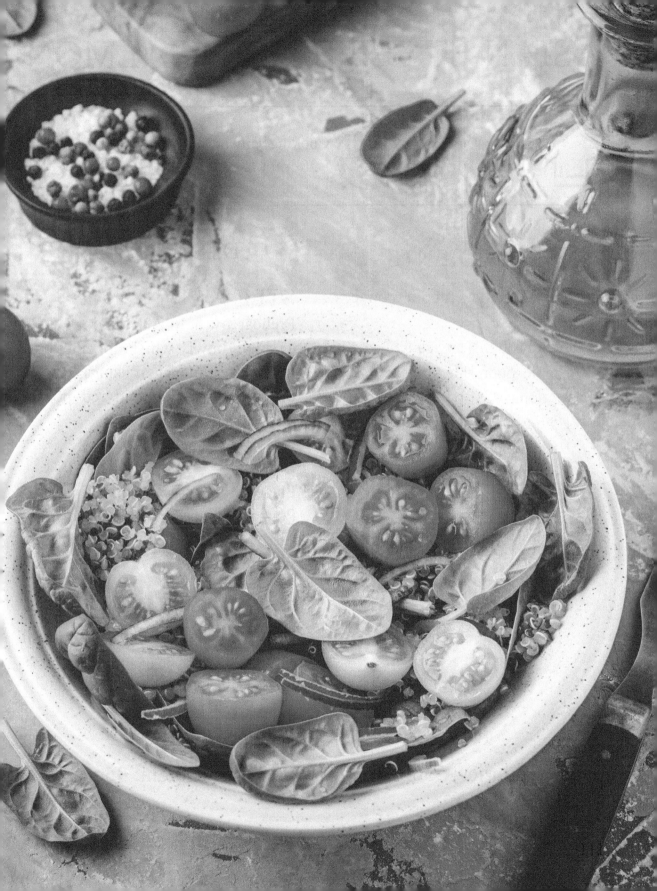

ASIAN-STYLE BAKED SALMON

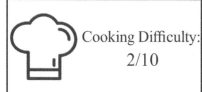 Cooking Difficulty: 2/10	 Cooking Time: 20 minutes	Servings: 4

INGREDIENTS

- 4 salmon fillets (about 6 ounces each)
- ¼ cup (60 ml) soy sauce
- 1 tablespoon rice vinegar (optional)
- 1 tablespoon sesame oil
- 1 teaspoon grated ginger
- 1 clove garlic, minced
- ½ teaspoon red pepper flakes
- 2 tablespoons sesame seeds
- green onions, for garnish (optional)

DESCRIPTION

STEP 1
Preheat oven to 400 degrees F. In a small bowl, whisk together soy sauce, rice vinegar (if using), sesame oil, ginger, garlic, and red pepper flakes.

STEP 2
Place salmon fillets in a baking dish. Pour marinade over salmon, making sure to coat evenly.Sprinkle with sesame seeds.

STEP 3
Bake for 15-20 minutes, or until salmon is cooked through and flakes easily with a fork. Serve immediately.

NUTRITIONAL INFORMATION

Calories: 350, Fat: 15g, Carbs: 5g, Protein: 35g

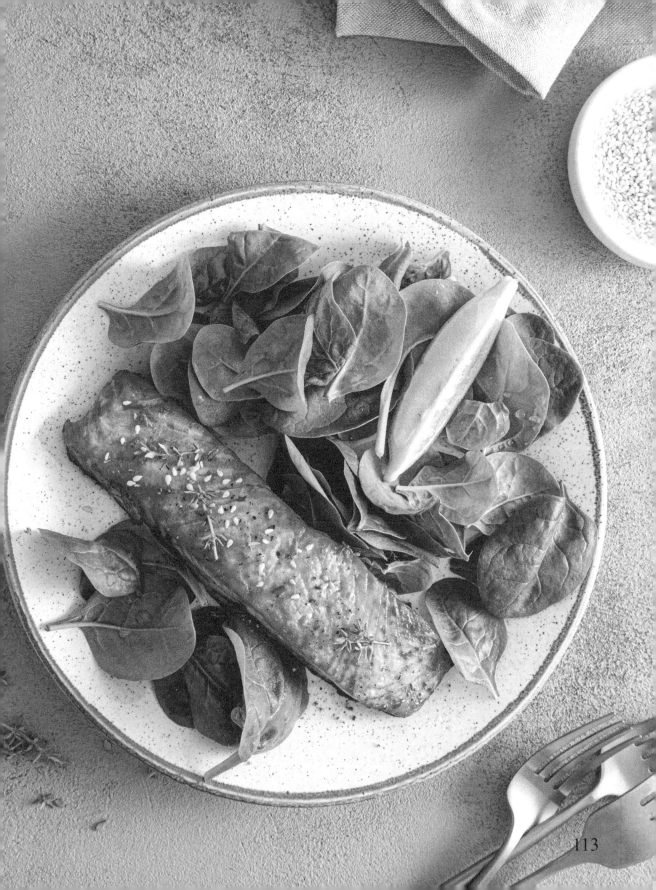

QUINOA STUFFED BELL PEPPERS

Cooking Difficulty: 2/10	Cooking Time: 24 minutes	Servings: 4

INGREDIENTS

- 4 large bell peppers, halved and seeds removed
- 1 cup quinoa, cooked
- 1 can (15 oz) black beans, drained and rinsed
- 1 cup corn kernels (fresh or frozen)
- 1 cup cherry tomatoes, halved
- 1/2 cup red onion, finely chopped
- 1/2 cup fresh cilantro, chopped
- 1 teaspoon cumin
- salt and pepper to taste
- 1 cup tomato sauce (for topping)

DESCRIPTION

STEP 1
In a large mixing bowl, combine cooked quinoa, black beans, corn, cherry tomatoes, red onion, cilantro, cumin, salt, and pepper. Mix well. Stuff each bell pepper half with the quinoa mixture.

STEP 2
Preheat the air fryer at 180°C. Place the stuffed bell peppers in the air fryer basket. Cook for 15-20 minutes until the peppers are tender.

NUTRITIONAL INFORMATION
Calories 295, Fat 8 g, Carbs 11 g, Protein 9 g

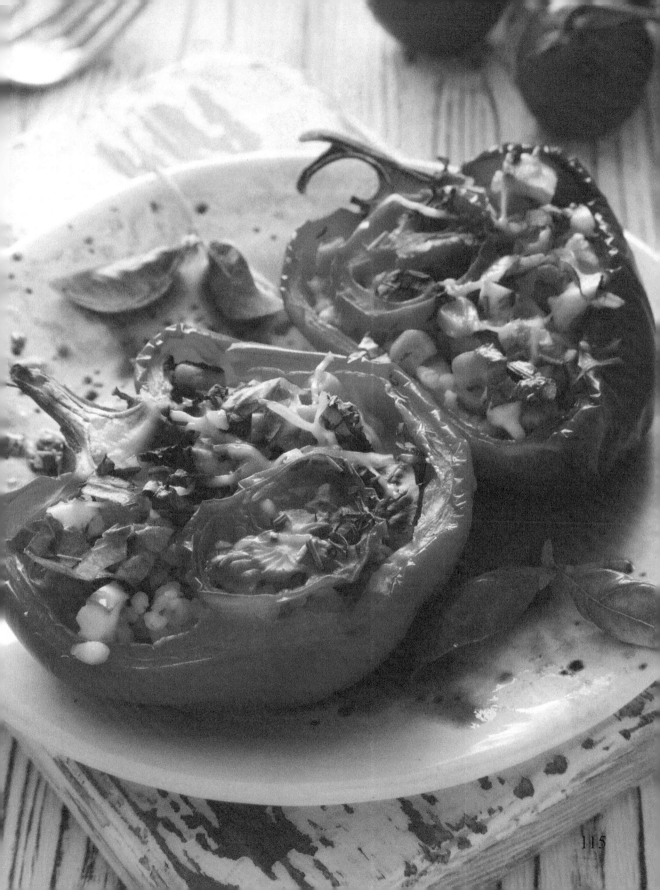

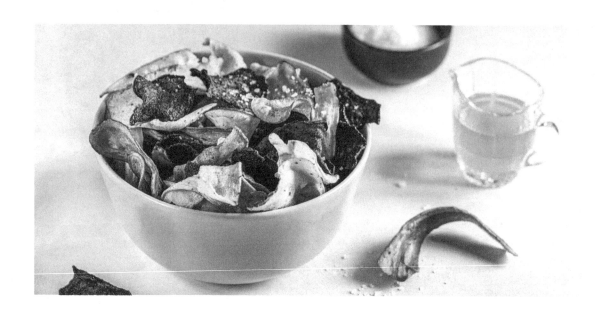

SNACKS & DESSERTS

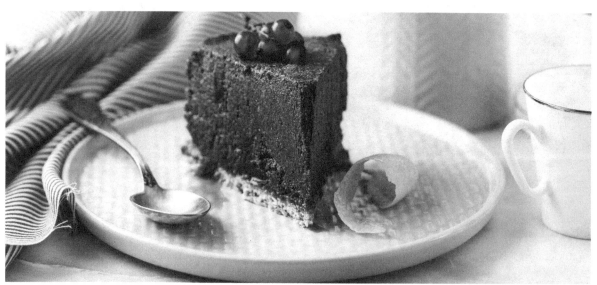

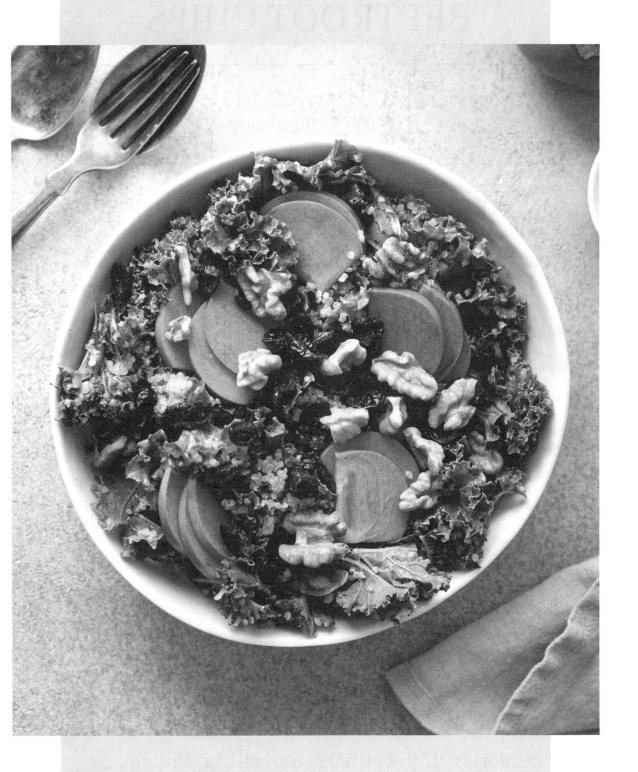

BEETROOT CHIPS

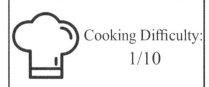 Cooking Difficulty: 1/10	 Cooking Time: 30 minutes	Servings: 4

INGREDIENTS

- 2 large beets (about 1 pound)
- 2 tablespoons olive oil
- 1 teaspoon salt
- 1/2 teaspoon black pepper
- 1/4 teaspoon paprika (optional)

DESCRIPTION

STEP 1
Preheat oven to 350 degrees F (180 degrees C). Wash and peel the beets thoroughly. Use a mandoline or vegetable slicer to thinly slice the beets.

STEP 2
In a large bowl, toss the beet slices with olive oil, salt, pepper, and paprika (optional). Arrange the beet slices in a single layer on a baking sheet lined with parchment paper.

STEP 3
Bake for 20-25 minutes, flipping the chips once halfway through, until they are crispy.

NUTRITIONAL INFORMATION

Calories: 150, Fat: 10g, Carbs: 15g, Protein: 3g

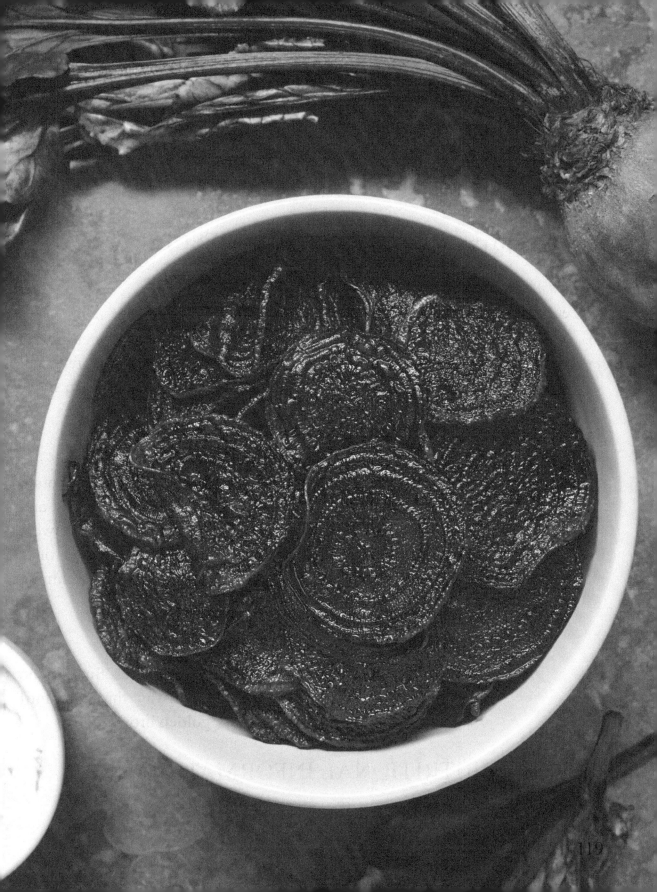

ROASTED SWEET POTATO

 Cooking Difficulty: 1/10

 Cooking Time: 30 minutes

 Servings: 2

INGREDIENTS

- 4 salmon fillets (about 6 ounces each)
- ¼ cup (60 ml) soy sauce
- 1 tablespoon rice vinegar (optional)
- 1 tablespoon sesame oil
- 1 teaspoon grated ginger
- 1 clove garlic, minced
- ½ teaspoon red pepper flakes
- 2 tablespoons sesame seeds
- green onions, for garnish (optional)

DESCRIPTION

STEP 1
Preheat oven to 400 degrees F. Wash and scrub the sweet potato thoroughly. Use a sharp knife to cut the sweet potato crosswise into slices about 1/2-inch thick.

STEP 2
In a large bowl, toss the sweet potato slices with olive oil, salt, pepper, and paprika (optional). Arrange the sweet potato slices in a single layer on a baking sheet lined with parchment paper.

STEP 3
Roast for 20-25 minutes, flipping the slices once halfway through, until tender and golden brown.

NUTRITIONAL INFORMATION

Calories: 200, Fat: 8g, Carbs: 10g, Protein: 4g

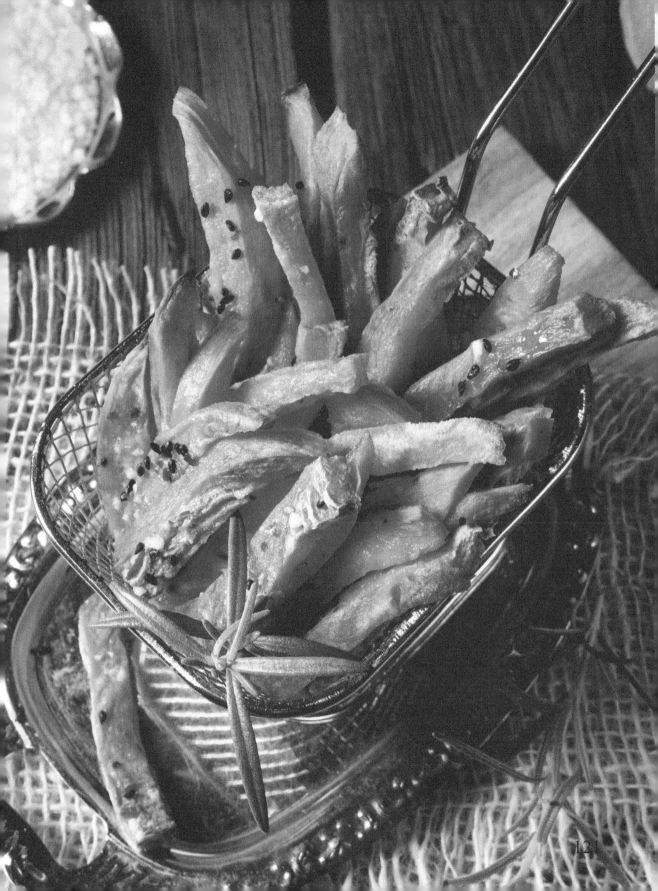

BROCCOLI HUMMUS

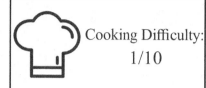 Cooking Difficulty: 1/10

 Cooking Time: 8 minutes

 Servings: 2

INGREDIENTS

- cup broccoli florets
- ½ cup canned chickpeas (or ½ cup cooked chickpeas)
- 2 tablespoons tahini
- 1 tablespoon olive oil
- 1 clove garlic
- juice of ½ lemon
- salt and pepper to taste
- 1 tablespoon water (optional)
- garnish: olive oil, paprika, parsley

DESCRIPTION

STEP 1
Bring a pot of salted water to a boil. Add the broccoli florets and cook for 2-3 minutes, until tender.

STEP 2
In a blender or food processor, combine the broccoli, chickpeas, tahini, olive oil, garlic, lemon juice, salt, and pepper. Blend until smooth.

STEP 3
If needed, add 1 tablespoon of water to make the hummus thinner. Transfer the hummus to a bowl and garnish with olive oil, paprika, and parsley.

NUTRITIONAL INFORMATION

Calories: 250, Fat: 15g, Carbs: 5g, Protein: 10g

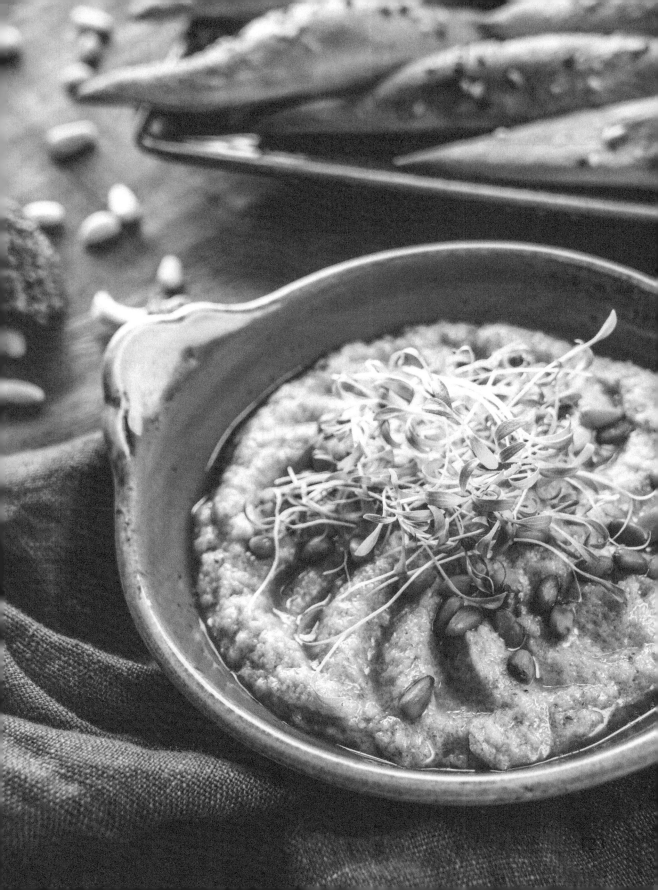

ALMOND MILK AND BLACKBERRY SMOOTHIE

 Cooking Difficulty: 1/10

 Cooking Time: 2 minutes

 Servings: 1

INGREDIENTS

- 1 cup unsweetened almond milk (or other plant-based milk)
- 1/2 cup frozen blackberries
- 1 banana
- 1 tablespoon chia seeds (optional)
- 1 tablespoon almond butter (optional)
- honey or agave syrup to taste (optional)

DESCRIPTION

STEP 1
Combine all ingredients in a blender and blend until smooth.

STEP 2
Enjoy! You can drink the smoothie immediately or chill it in the refrigerator before drinking.

NUTRITIONAL INFORMATION

Calories: 300, Fat: 15g, Carbs: 40g, Protein: 10g

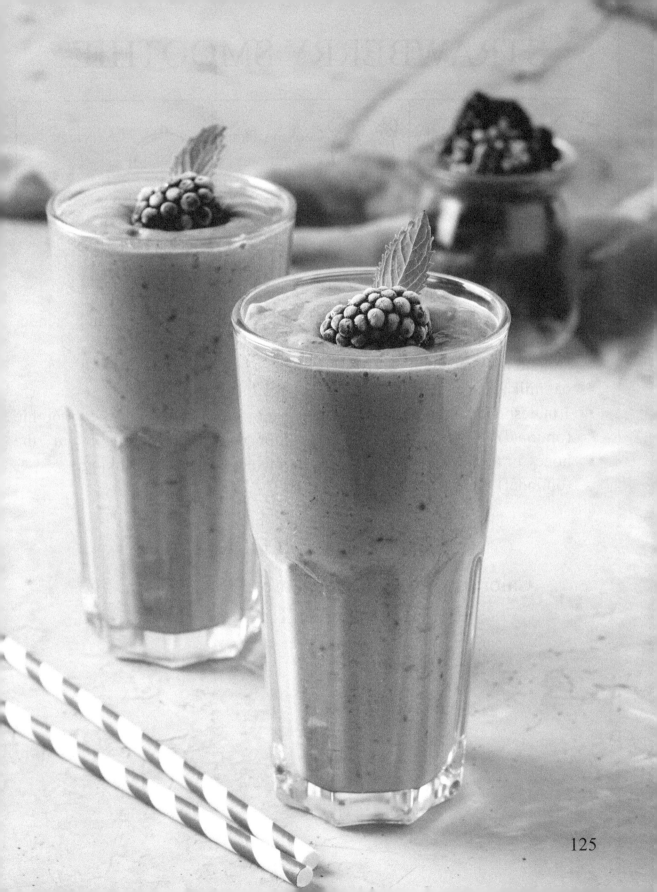

STRAWBERRY SMOOTHIE

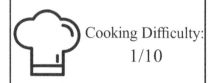 Cooking Difficulty: 1/10

 Cooking Time: 2 minutes

 Servings: 1

INGREDIENTS

- 1 cup frozen strawberries
- 1 banana
- 1 cup plant-based milk (such as almond milk, coconut milk, or oat milk)
- 1 tablespoon almond butter (optional)
- honey or agave syrup to taste (optional)

DESCRIPTION

STEP 1
Combine all ingredients in a blender and blend until smooth.

STEP 2
Enjoy! You can drink the smoothie immediately or chill it in the refrigerator before drinking.

NUTRITIONAL INFORMATION
Calories: 350, Fat: 15g, Carbs: 35g, Protein: 5g

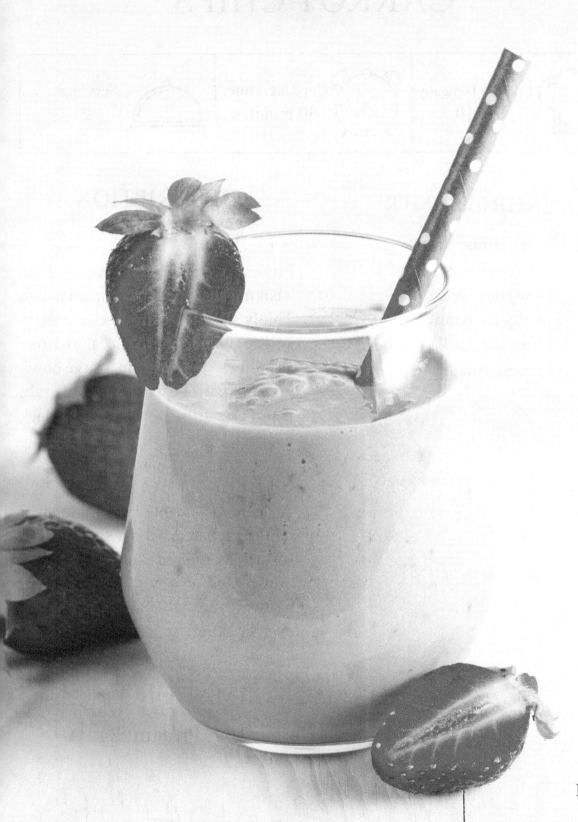

CARROT CHIPS

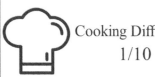 Cooking Difficulty: 1/10	Cooking Time: 30 minutes	Servings: 2

INGREDIENTS

- 2 large carrots
- 1 tablespoon olive oil
- 1/2 teaspoon salt
- 1/4 teaspoon paprika
- 1/4 teaspoon garlic powder
- 1/8 teaspoon black pepper

DESCRIPTION

STEP 1

Preheat oven to 350 degrees F. Line a baking sheet with parchment paper. Thinly slice the carrots. Use a sharp knife or mandoline to slice the carrots as thinly as possible. In a large bowl, toss the carrots with olive oil, salt, paprika, garlic powder, and black pepper.

STEP 2

Arrange the carrots in a single layer on the prepared baking sheet. Bake for 15-20 minutes, or until golden brown and crispy. Flip the chips halfway through baking to ensure even cooking.

NUTRITIONAL INFORMATION

Calories: 150, Fat: 5g, Carbs: 10g, Protein: 2g

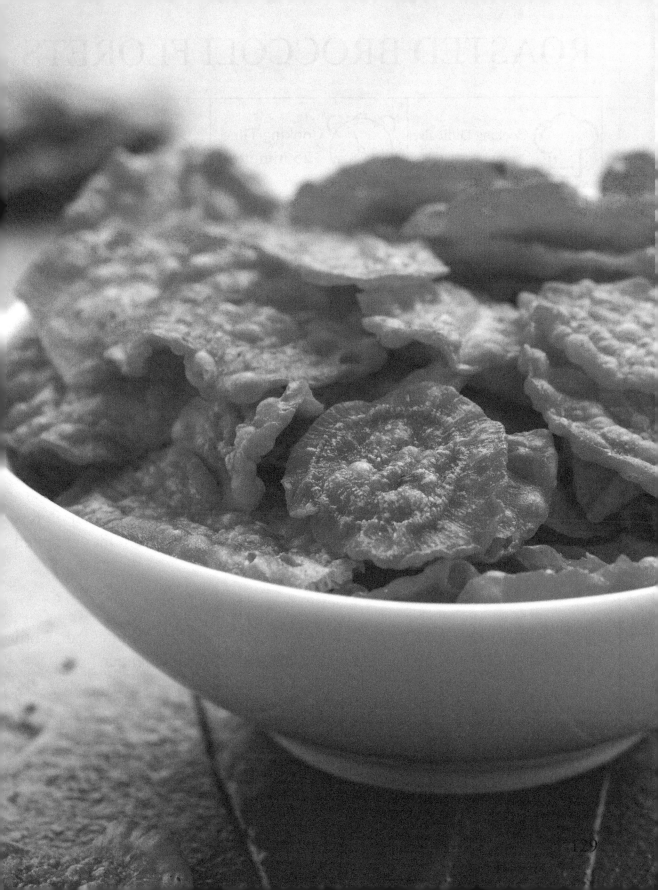

ROASTED BROCCOLI FLORETS

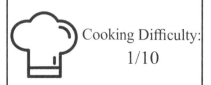 Cooking Difficulty: 1/10

 Cooking Time: 25 minutes

 Servings: 2

INGREDIENTS

- 2 cups broccoli florets
- 1 tablespoon olive oil
- 1/2 teaspoon salt
- 1/4 teaspoon black pepper
- 1/4 teaspoon paprika
- 1/4 teaspoon garlic powder
- pinch of red pepper flakes (optional)

DESCRIPTION

STEP 1
Preheat oven to 400 degrees F (200 degrees C). Line a baking sheet with parchment paper.

STEP 2
In a large bowl, toss broccoli florets with olive oil, salt, pepper, paprika, garlic powder, and red pepper flakes (optional). Arrange broccoli florets in a single layer on the prepared baking sheet.

STEP 3
Roast for 15-20 minutes, or until golden brown and tender.

NUTRITIONAL INFORMATION

Calories: 100, Fat: 5g, Carbs: 10g, Protein: 3g

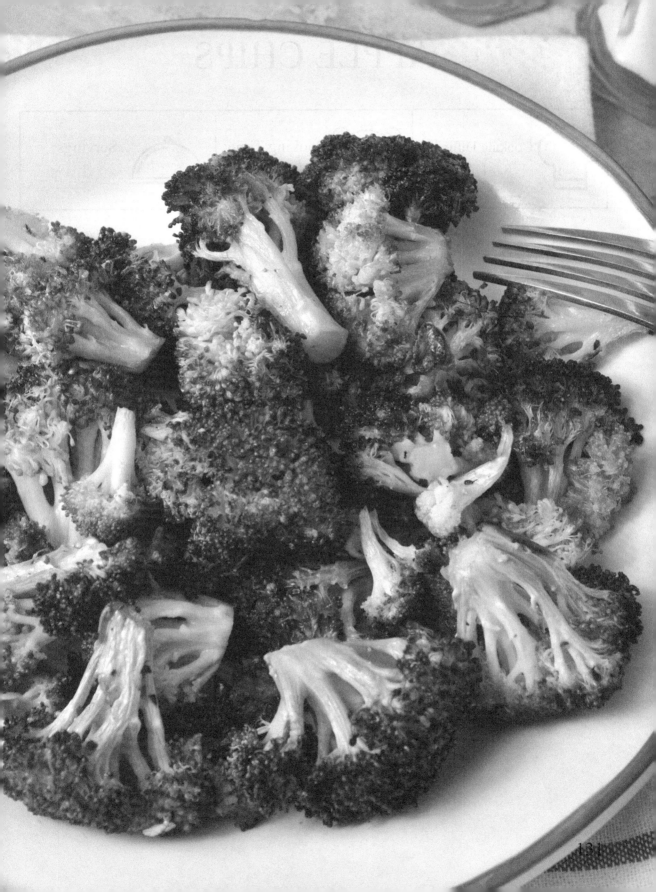

APPLE CHIPS

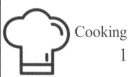 Cooking Difficulty: 1/10

 Cooking Time: 120 minutes

 Servings: 2

INGREDIENTS

- 2 large apples (sweet varieties)
- 1 tablespoon lemon juice (optional)
- 1/2 teaspoon cinnamon (optional)
- 1/4 teaspoon nutmeg (optional)

DESCRIPTION

STEP 1
Slice apples thinly. Drizzle with lemon juice (optional).

STEP 2
Add spices (cinnamon, nutmeg - to taste).

STEP 3
Arrange in a single layer on a parchment-lined baking sheet.

STEP 4
Bake at 200°F (100°C) for 1-2 hours until crispy. Cool and enjoy!

NUTRITIONAL INFORMATION

Calories: 150, Fat: 3g, Carbs: 10g, Protein: 1g

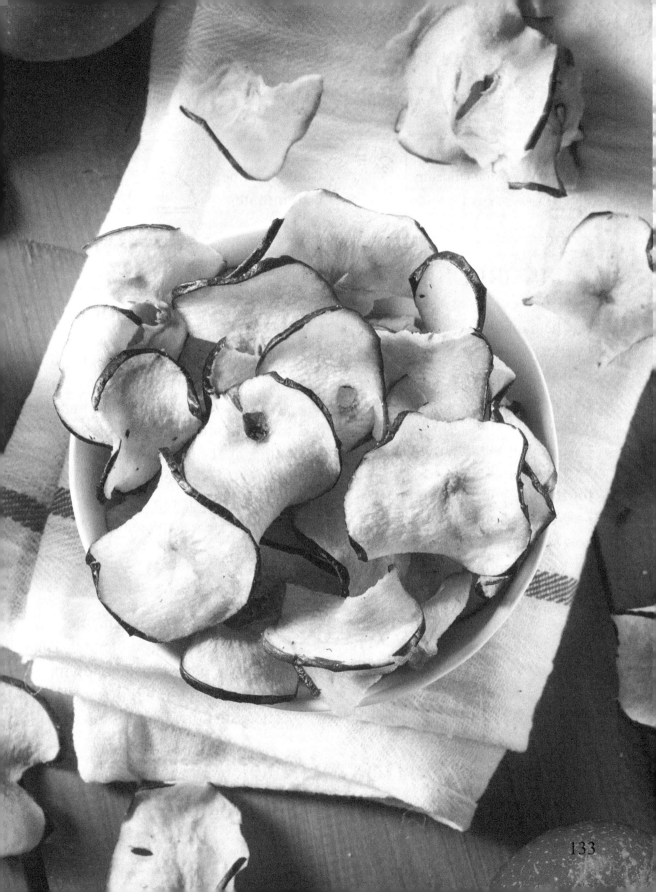

PANNA COTTA WITH STRAWBERRY COMPOTE

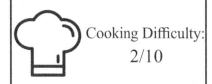 Cooking Difficulty: 2/10

 Cooking Time: 10 minutes

 Servings: 2

INGREDIENTS

for the panna cotta:
- 2 cups canned coconut milk
- 1/2 cup vegan yogurt
- 1/4 cup maple syrup, or to taste
- 1 teaspoon vanilla extract
- 1/2 teaspoon agar-agar powder
- 1/4 teaspoon salt

for the strawberry compote:
- 2 cups fresh strawberries
- 1/4 cup maple syrup, or to taste
- 1 tablespoon lemon juice

DESCRIPTION

STEP 1
Combine coconut milk, yogurt, maple syrup, vanilla extract, agar-agar, and salt in a saucepan over medium heat. Bring to a boil, whisking constantly, until agar-agar dissolves. Remove from heat and let cool slightly. Pour into 4 small ramekins or glasses. Refrigerate for at least 4 hours, or until set.

STEP 2
Combine strawberries, maple syrup, and lemon juice in a blender. Blend until smooth. Refrigerate for 30 minutes to chill. Top each panna cotta with strawberry compote.

NUTRITIONAL INFORMATION
Calories: 180, Fat: 8g, Carbs: 10g, Protein: 5g

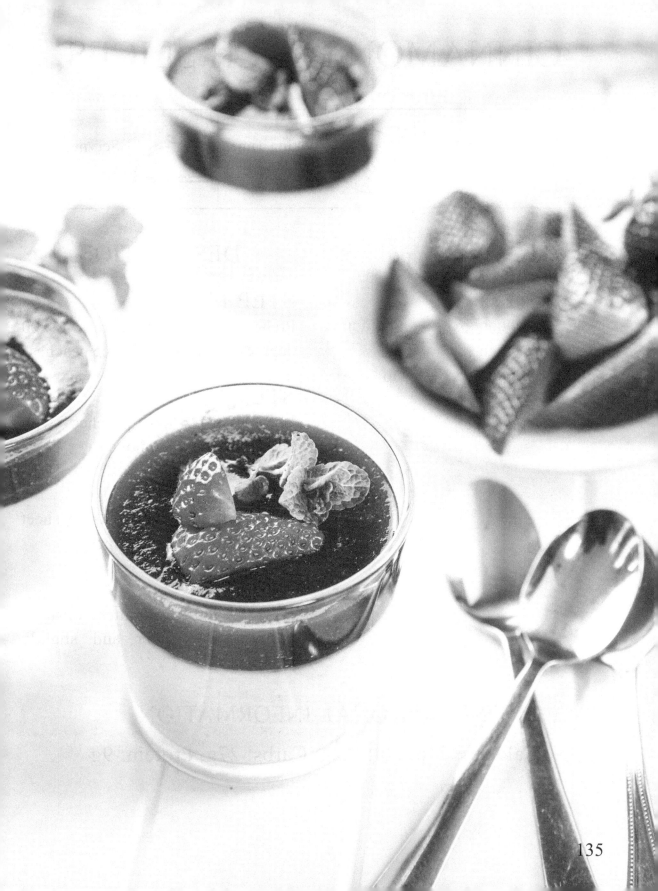

CINNAMON PEACH SLICES

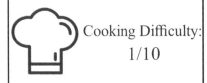 Cooking Difficulty: 1/10

 Cooking Time: 30 minutes

 Servings: 2

INGREDIENTS

- 2 peaches
- 1/2 teaspoon ground cinnamon
- 1/4 teaspoon salt
- 1 tablespoon honey (or to taste)

DESCRIPTION

STEP 1
Preheat oven to 400 degrees F (200 degrees C). Wash and slice peaches.

STEP 2
In a bowl, toss peaches with cinnamon, salt, and honey.

STEP 3
Arrange peaches on a baking sheet lined with parchment paper.

STEP 4
Bake for 20-25 minutes, or until peaches are tender and slightly browned.

NUTRITIONAL INFORMATION
Calories: 216, Fat: 8.2g, Carbs: 27g, Protein: 9g

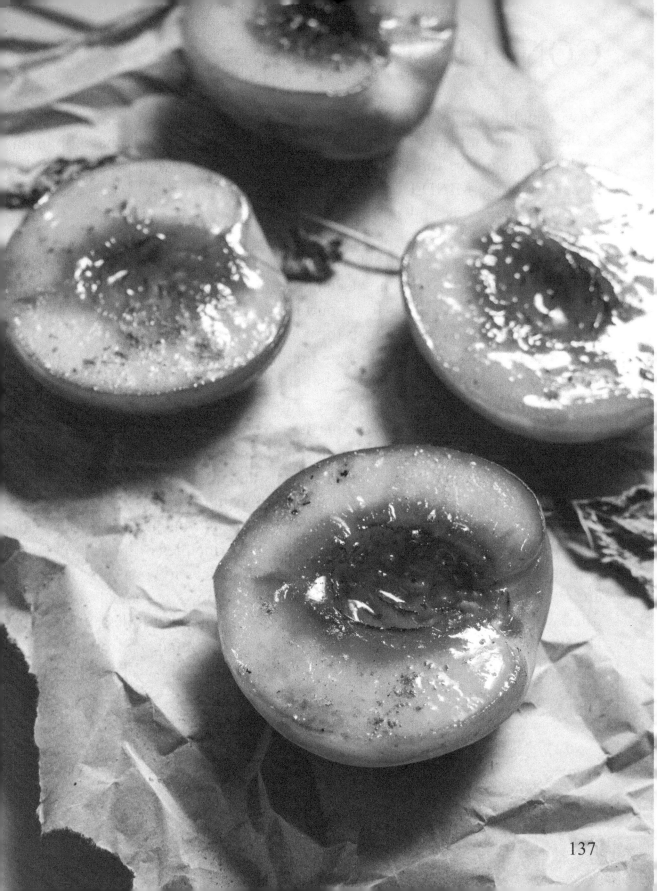

CONCLUSION

As we conclude our journey through the MIND Diet Cookbook, we are reminded of the profound impact that nutrition, lifestyle, and mindset can have on brain health and cognitive function. Throughout these pages, we have explored the principles of the MIND Diet, delved into the science behind its efficacy, and discovered delicious and nutritious recipes to support our journey towards optimal brain health.

In today's fast-paced world, where cognitive decline and neurodegenerative diseases loom as significant threats, empowering ourselves with knowledge and adopting proactive measures to support brain health is more crucial than ever. The MIND Diet offers a roadmap for nourishing our brains with the nutrients they need to thrive, while also promoting healthy habits and lifestyle choices that enhance cognitive vitality and resilience.

As you embark on your MIND Diet journey, remember that small changes can yield significant results. Whether it's swapping out processed snacks for nutrient-rich alternatives, incorporating more fruits and vegetables into your meals, or engaging in regular physical activity and mindfulness practices, every step you take towards prioritizing brain health matters.

Let this book serve as a guide and inspiration as you navigate your path towards lifelong brain health. By embracing the principles of the MIND Diet, cultivating healthy habits, and making mindful choices in your daily life, you are investing in a future where cognitive vitality knows no bounds—a future filled with clarity, resilience, and the joy of living life to the fullest.

Here's to nourishing your brain, empowering your mind, and embracing a future of limitless possibilities. Cheers to your health and well-being!

Stella Harper

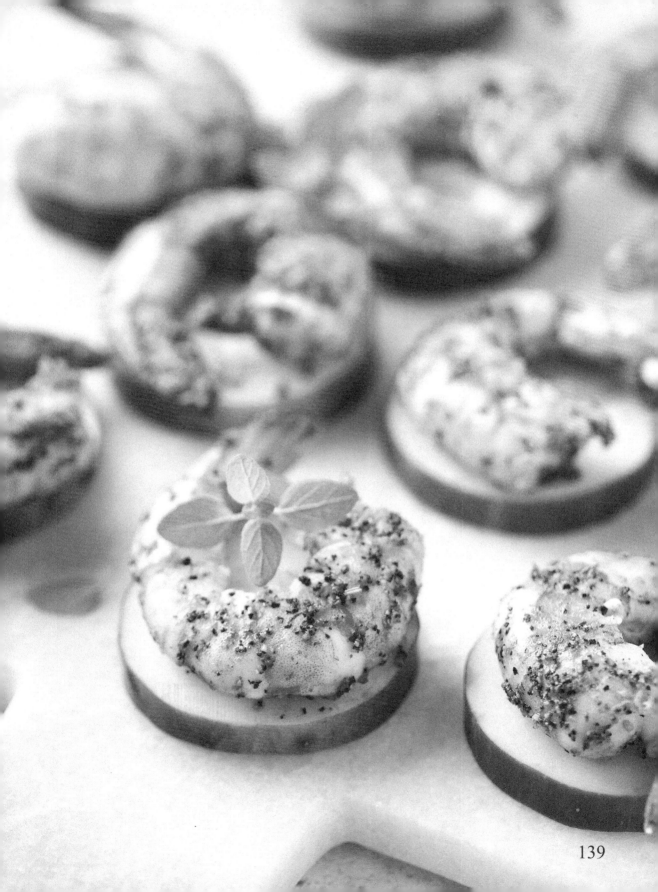

Made in the USA
Monee, IL
28 September 2024

66833992R00077